# Taking Charge
of
# Your Health

# Taking Charge
## of
# Your Health

Understanding the System Could Save Your Life
A Practical Guide to Getting Better Medical Care

- Get the Most from Your Doctors
- Stay Sane When Dealing with Insurance Issues
- Access Your Medical Records
- Obtain Other Opinions
- Manage Your Medications So They Don't Kill You
- Put Your Wellness Team Together
- Get Information
- Survive Your Hospital Stays and Treatments

Alice Hodge
and
Mary Lonergan

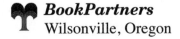
***BookPartners***
Wilsonville, Oregon

## Disclaimer

In this book, we share our own insights and experiences gained as patients. We are not trained in the medical or counseling fields. Our recommendations and those of other patients included in this book are not to be taken as a substitute for professional advice. It is important that you communicate and work with your own healthcare professionals with regard to your medical care.

***BookPartners, Inc.***
P.O. Box 922
Wilsonville, Oregon 97070

*To Jim and Dick, who have been there for us in the best and worst of times.*

# Acknowledgments

First and foremost, we want to thank Steve Carr, without whose encouragement and guidance this book would not have been written.

So many have given so much to turn this effort into a reality. Some have shared their firsthand experience, expertise or knowledge. Others have given us valuable feedback on our manuscript. Still others have played a critical role in helping with the production of the book. Our heartfelt thanks go to Jodi Austin, Nancy Boughey, Doris Cohen, Anne Halsted, Jim Hodge, Barbara Hoffer, Mary Horvers, Sarah Iaia, Anne Keyser, Dr. J. J. Keyser, Dr. Detlef Kutzscher, Dr. Jeff Lindenbaum, Dick Lonergan, Marjorie Lonergan, Pam McAllister, Theresa McCrea, Sally McGeoch, Ann Nutting, Bill Nutting, Lee Olivier, Dr. Robert Rodvien, Stephanie Ralphs, Bambi Schwartz, Dr. Diane Scott, Dr. Paul H. Sugarbaker, Ginger Sulpizio, Dr. Lenore Terr, Dr. Clay Thomson, Dr. Debu Tripathy, Mary Lou Whitcomb and Wells Whitney.

We are also grateful to the Community Health Resource Center, California Pacific Medical Center, Hospice of Marin, Planetree Library, The Institute for Health and Healing, UCSF/Mount Zion Medical Center and The Health Library at Stanford Shopping Center.

Last, but certainly not least, we want to thank our families, close friends and each other for putting up with the process.

*"That which does not kill me makes me stronger."*

Friedrich Nietzsche

# Table of Contents

# Worksheets and Sample Questions

(Worksheets and Sample Questions can be copied at 150 percent to fit on standard 8-1/2" x 11" paper.)

# Foreword

## Why We Wrote This Book

*For several months, I had been in and out of the hospital because of chest pain. Despite several angioplasties and a pacemaker implant, I continued to be plagued by increasing pain and shortness of breath. Although I was clearly having trouble, my doctors did not believe that my problems were heart-related, because my most recent test results did not indicate typical angina.*

*The worse my symptoms got, the lower my spirits sank. The days, weeks and months it took to get to the root of my problem not only drained me physically and emotionally, but also left me scared to death. I went from outgoing and upbeat to constantly depressed and increasingly withdrawn from family and friends. I felt like a burden to everyone and I dreaded calling my doctors or going to the emergency room, for fear they would not believe me. I lost faith in myself, which only made me feel worse. After countless trips to the emergency room and six hospital admissions within one year, a friend introduced me to Mary and Alice. They taught me the skills I needed to take charge of my situation, and helped me change my life. Today, although I continue to have difficulties, I have developed a better working relationship with my doctors and a much more positive outlook for myself as I learn to live with heart disease.*

Joyce

We first met as neighbors living in San Francisco. We were two happily married women living successful lives: Mary, mother of two young children and owner of a thriving catering business, and Alice, a fast-rising executive in the corporate world. Everything in our lives seemed right. Little did we know how quickly our realities would change.

Alice was twenty-six years old when her ovarian problems began. Mary was just thirty-six when she was diagnosed with lymphoma. For the last sixteen years we both have been on a roller coaster ride — diagnoses followed by treatments, followed by high hopes of recovery, followed by the discovery of new symptoms of disease.

Collectively, we survived repeated bouts with four different types of cancer, one major heart crisis and the full gamut of surgeries, radiation, chemotherapies, tests, medications, life style modification therapies, adjunctive and alternative treatment programs, depression cycles, and the stubborn side effects and general misery that go with all of the above.

Neither of us set out to write a book, but we wanted to help people in similar situations profit from our experiences. After talking with many other survivors of serious illness, we conducted a series of workshops at the Community Health Resource Center in San Francisco. Finally we put our hard-earned knowledge down on paper in order to acquaint you with the process of organization, communication and research that will aid you to better understand and direct your own medical care. By utilizing a few simple skills, we have been able to take charge of the decisions affecting our treatment, which in turn made us feel more positive about our situations. At first we were afraid that we might not have enough material to fill the pages of a book. How wrong we were! The moment we started to write, words flowed with the speed of a rushing river, and at times it was almost impossible to keep up.

Our intention in sharing our experiences is neither to recap the tragedies of our lives nor to pontificate about our views on the entire medical system. Frankly, we don't have the time or energy for either. What we want to accomplish is to guide you through the healthcare maze in the event that you are faced with a serious medical challenge. We do not have medical degrees; neither one of us is a doctor, psychotherapist or social worker, but we have become experts at successfully getting through crises and getting on with the joy of living life.

Had a book like this been available at the time our health problems started, we would have greatly appreciated it. It would have smoothed out the rough road a patient has to walk to combat illness. Will this book provide you with all the answers you need? Probably not — but hey — what we've learned got us this far. We are all on our own journeys. No one can take the walk for us. You must blaze your own trail.

By sharing our firsthand knowledge, we will provide you with a practical guide through the maze of doctor visits, tests, treatments and hospital stays, as well as the emotional upheaval of your new, post-diagnosis life. We have also included a number of anecdotes to help you learn from the shared experiences of others who have walked this road before you.

From all we are presenting in this book, use what works and don't fret that your way may be different from ours. It is our wish that the information in this book will help you take charge of your health and ease the path to getting well.

The Authors

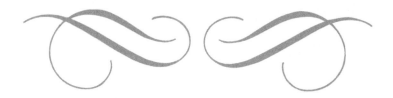

# Chapter One

# Diagnosis and Discovery

*My doctor entered the examination room. I was there for a follow-up visit, because he had spotted "some things" on a previous exam and had run a couple of additional tests. "Nothing to worry about," he had said as we parted company the week before.*

*"Well, we may have a problem," he said, gently. "I'm not absolutely sure what it is, but I think that we should go in and take a look."*

*"Okay," I responded, not wanting to appear overly concerned. "Let me talk with my husband and get back to you. How soon would you book the surgery?"*

*"Next week," he said.*

*I don't remember driving my car, but somehow I ended up back at my office. The phone rang. I talked for a while and shuffled the papers on my desk. All of a sudden, tears came in a flood. As they streamed down my face, I turned to the wall but I couldn't see a thing. Oh my God, I thought. I'm thirty-eight years old, I'm seriously ill and I have to go to the hospital. What's happening to me?*

Alice

## Get Ready to Face Your Situation

Let's face it. It doesn't matter how life has treated you up to now. Regardless of your education, your status in the community, or your personal situation, when you are diagnosed with a serious illness, your world is forever changed.

Whether the news comes unexpectedly, like a shot out of the blue, or following months of dealing with troubling symptoms and endless visits to the doctor, it hits you like a punch in the stomach. In some cases it may take you a while to realize what the doctor has said. In others you may even breathe a sigh of relief to finally have a "name" that legitimizes your complaints. At least they can't call you crazy anymore. Whatever the circumstances leading up to your diagnosis, the shock and bewilderment you feel when told that you have a serious health problem ultimately makes you feel worse for the knowing. You may experience anger, confusion, guilt, sadness, fear or denial. These are all perfectly normal emotions.

What can you do? What are you supposed to think? What is going to happen — to you, and to those who love and depend upon you? These worries and more fill every corner of your mind — constantly. Often, you can't eat, think straight or get to sleep, because there are so many unanswered questions and "what ifs." Add to that physically not feeling well and your situation goes from worse to unbearable. Not only are you sick, but you feel as though your life is spinning out of control.

When the disease is first identified, just trying to understand the meaning and implications of your diagnosis requires so much energy and emotion that developing a thoughtful plan of action seems nearly impossible. You may feel like pulling the covers over your head and hoping that, when you wake up again, this will simply have been a bad dream.

Nothing in your experience has prepared you for this untimely turn of events. Life up to now may have been normal. You may even have prided yourself on your resourcefulness or your ability to adapt to tough situations. But when you come face to face with a serious illness, your "instincts" often suddenly stop functioning; your "inner sense of what to do" no longer transmits any helpful messages. From one moment to the next you feel as though you are on a carnival Tilt-A-Whirl, standing strapped to the wall while the ride spins you around — and then the floor drops out. In one split second, you go from being a "normal person" to being a patient, and the shock of this sudden change in status may cause you to lose sight of the strengths and skills that, until now, allowed you to operate successfully in your everyday world.

If your disease turns out to be life-threatening, you may be urged to act quickly. The pressure, both internal and external, to do something is intense. In some cases, there may be little known or written about your illness or its treatment possibilities. Usually, however, there are a wealth of information and several treatment options available for you to consider.

Your first concern is to gain a clear understanding of how to proceed. How can you instantly acquire the resources and acumen needed to make the right decisions? Where do you begin? As you stagger off of the carnival ride, you find that your legs don't work, you can't walk straight, and your world keeps spinning around you.

As patients diagnosed with life-threatening illnesses, we too were overwhelmed by the same issues and dilemmas you now face. We also saw others deal with the same problems. Eventually, in the process of confronting our own diseases, we learned how to equip ourselves with the means and the mindset necessary to choose our own paths on the road to wellness. Let us guide you. Allow us to teach you some simple steps that will help you gain control of your situation and allow you to make good decisions regarding your care. We want to help you avoid the feelings of desperation that can easily lead to depression and increasingly ill health.

By making an effort to gain control of your situation and by taking the time to incorporate some simple steps into your approach, you will be better equipped to make good decisions regarding your healthcare. As a result, you will develop a more positive sense of yourself and your situation.

# Chapter Two

# Take Charge

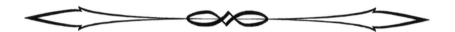

*I was blessed with a strong constitution, good genes and great luck. I hardly ever got sick. So even when I saw a large, white lump staring back at me from the magnetic resonance imaging test (MRI), I didn't believe it was anything to be concerned about.*

*Several weeks before, on a business trip to Stockholm, Sweden, I had found myself staggering down the street bumping into lamp posts, even before my first cocktail. I was worried, but I attributed my problem to jet lag.*

*I mentioned my experience to my wife when I returned home, which quickly led to a visit with our general practitioner, followed by an MRI, a follow-up visit, and finally a trip to the offices of the leading brain tumor specialist at U.C. Medical Center in San Francisco.*

*I liked the specialist. He was quiet, thoughtful, and a fellow scientist. We examined the abnormalities present in the MRI and discussed his findings with scientific detachment. Suddenly it hit me — this was my head we were talking about; the shadows on the X-ray indicated an acoustic neuroma on my brain; and it was my brain that he wanted to cut open. It was then that feelings of panic and fear set in. Yes, I had to admit fear!*

Wells

## First Things First — The *What* Stage

The period immediately after you have been told that something is wrong is truly horrible. In our cases, we didn't even know specifically what our problems were at first. It is precisely this feeling of not knowing that makes your situation almost unbearable.

There is no magic antidote for these feelings of uncertainty. Though easier said than done, our best advice is to try to remain calm about your situation. Much like a baby who is learning to walk, you must get your balance and begin to put one foot in front of the other. No matter how fast you once were able to run in life, coping with a serious illness sets you back to your first steps. Just like a baby, you must first learn how to stand and then to walk in this new world before you attempt to run again.

## Getting It Down on Paper

The first step in the process of gaining control of your medical condition is to write down exactly what you understand about it. Start by taking two pieces of paper and placing them side by side in front of you. On one sheet, list everything you already know about your situation. Be prepared to discover that your effort will raise more questions than it answers. That's okay. Getting your questions answered is also part of the process. On the second sheet, write all of the questions and concerns that come to mind. For example:

- When did I first become aware of a problem?
- What did the doctor call what I have?
- How did she describe it to me?
- Is it caused by anything definite?
- If so, is it hereditary? Environmental? Behavioral?
- What is the recommended treatment? What are my alternatives?

- What are my chances of being cured?
- What are my chances of a recurrence?
- How long will I be sick?

No matter how long your two lists become, keep writing until everything you can think of is recorded. Your primary goals are to assess what you *do* know at this point and to get all of your apprehensions and questions out of your head and onto paper. As long as your questions are spinning around in your head, all they do is worry and bewilder you. Writing everything down accomplishes three important objectives:

- It allows you to relax (somewhat).
- It reminds you what you need to ask your doctor, your insurance company or others who will be involved in your treatment.
- It becomes the basis for your action plan.

As your questions are answered in the days and weeks to come, you will learn more about the nature of your disease, you will expand your vocabulary to include many new technical or scientific words that describe your condition, and you will begin to understand the options that are available to you. Little did you realize when you started on this journey that not only would you get the equivalent of a new education, but you would also need to learn a new language!

*In the weeks following my diagnosis, I absorbed information like a sponge. I listened to everything my well-meaning friends said and I read whatever was shoved into my hands. Halfway through this process, the absurdity of trying to acquire a full medical education on my cancer in three weeks finally hit home. I decided what I really needed was a working vocabulary, up-to-date treatment information, and a medical team who would answer my questions. Only then could I trust the doctors enough to proceed with treatment. I still had lots of questions, but at least I could tolerate the unknowns.*

Mary Frances

The following examples show what your information and question sheets might look like. Don't just use the exact forms we have provided. Adapt them to fit your specific situation.

## Understanding My Medical Condition

My problem is

The medical term for my condition is

My condition is caused by or the result of

The symptoms and manifestations of my condition are

The most medically accepted treatment method is

Other treatment methods are

My long-term prognosis is

Other information I know about my condition

Recommended lifestyle changes are

# Questions I Have about My Medical Condition

What in layman's terms does *(cardiomyopathy)* mean?

What specifically is *(ascites),* and how does it relate to my diagnosis?

What are the possible causes of my disease?

Do other family members have it? If so, why?

Are there possible environmental causes? What are they?

Are there possible lifestyle causes? Why?

I know that I have *(colon cancer),* but what specifically is causing me to have so many digestive problems?

I know that I have a *(heart condition),* but why does that mean that my fingers are sometimes numb?

Does going through treatment mean that I will be cured? If not, why not?

Don't be discouraged if you aren't able to fill in many of the blanks on the Understanding My Medical Condition page or if you have loads of questions on your second sheet. Remember, this exercise is a process of discovery. Part of your discovery is coming to terms with what you already know and what you still need to learn. Your questions will guide your search for greater understanding; they will show you what further steps you need to take; and they will help you see what to do next.

## The Next Step

Just like the baby who is learning to walk, consider yourself ready to make the transition from knees first to feet first. Your next steps are to identify what are the best ways for you to go about getting your questions answered and who are the people best able to help. You can work on this alone, but this is a good time to ask a spouse, friends or other loved ones to help you. Often people close to you want to help in whatever ways they can, but they are uncomfortable about initiating the effort. By reaching out to them with a specific request, you can bridge that gulf. Reaching out also helps to ensure that their efforts on your behalf are focused in ways that are meaningful and beneficial to you. (We go into the subject of personal dynamics in greater detail in chapter 7.)

Approach your search with an attitude of adventure and discovery. Make it an exercise in "creative brainstorming." Focus on possibilities, not on problems or implementation issues. For example, if you have breast cancer or diabetes, think about how you can learn more about your condition. You might make a note to get on the Internet or to contact national and/or local associations which focus on these diseases. You may even write down the names of people or places that you recall have been associated with your illness. Do *not*, however, obsess at this point about the details. The appropriate methods of discovery *will* come.

When you are ready, try to organize your possible avenues into groups and think about who you know who would be best equipped to search for answers. Who do you know who can help you to understand all of the different medical terms used to describe your disease and its treatment? Do you have a friend (or a friend of a friend) who is a nurse, doctor or medical researcher? How can you find out what resources the Internet has to offer? Perhaps this is a job for your sixteen-year-old son or niece. Are there any alternative or complementary therapies that you should consider at the same time you are looking into medical treatment options? Who do you know who can help you investigate these?

Do not be discouraged if, at first, this process doesn't seem to come easily for you. Remember, little Johnny didn't walk effortlessly the first time he tried to either. If it all gets too overwhelming, then stop for a while. Feel good about what you have accomplished, even if it was just one or two things. Little by little, and with help, you will see how to go about finding the answers to your questions. Your "to do" list may be long, but, with a little effort, your means for accomplishing it will seem boundless.

## A Word of Advice

Generally, we both adhere to the "now is as good a time as any" philosophy of life. With that in mind, it seems appropriate here for us to introduce to you what we will call a *pay-attention axiom:*

*No matter what worked best for you in your life before you were sick, know that, now, you are better off not traveling this new road alone.*

Some of you who live alone, or in lonely circumstances, may be honestly at a loss to think of who will help you in your new situation. This can itself be a devastating and depressing realization. The truth is, however, no one really has to be alone today. Depending upon where you live, there is generally a range of reasonably accessible community and religious based social service/help programs. And, if travelling to one of these is not practical, then pick up the telephone and call for assistance. More often than not, being alone is a state of mind, rather than a physical reality. We had one woman, who attended our seminar, insist that she was totally alone in the Bay Area and that there was no one available to help her. This came as a big surprise to her friend, who not only brought her to our session, but was seated right beside her while the woman was verbally lamenting about her lonely situation. As we discussed the subject in further depth, it turned out that our "lonely" woman not only volunteered each week at a senior citizens center but she had a daughter living in a nearby city! Sometimes, we must look beyond our assumptions of reality.

Think again of little Johnny learning to walk. Like him, you will be a lot more successful at it when someone is there to assist. Taking an active role in your treatment and care is important. Insisting, however, that you are all alone in this world or that no one else but you can do all of the things necessary for your recovery is short-sighted, arrogant and just plain stupid. In order for you to gain control over your health and well-being, you need to actively bring others into your life. This means even *asking* for help when need be.

This need for cooperative behavior can be especially difficult for those among us who are uncomfortable asking for help — or for those who feel best "doing for themselves." Our advice: *get over it!* You are better off giving up some control and increasing the prospects of getting well, than always needing to be in control, thereby decreasing your prospects of survival.

From a purely selfish point of view, you need to do this, so that you can focus all of your available resources on fighting your disease. Who knows, you may even be pleasantly surprised to realize that there are some people out there who are better at doing the things that you need done for you than you are!

From here on out, getting well depends less on being in control and more on maintaining a balance between the negative and positive factors affecting your physical and mental well-being. Let go of your need to control and you will find yourself more in control than you ever were before. As part of this, allow those who really care about you to help you achieve the recovery that you so desire.

If need be, think of yourself as the producer of a great movie in the making. Find an experienced director; have those who act best play their parts; allow the set and costume crews to establish the scene; let the musicians make the music; have the caterers satisfy your appetite; and you, taking in what everyone has to offer, craft the most beautiful image possible for yourself.

*Two things were most important to me during the weeks before my major operation. The first of these was under-standing all that I would be going through during the surgery and immediately beyond. And second was having an advocate — someone other than me who could make all of the calls, push the doctors, insurance company and hospital into making the right arrangements, and rally me to get my family and financial arrangements in order.*

*My wife was wonderful filling this role. She brought to the challenge the right mix of skepticism (about systems) and optimism (about my prospects) along with plenty of "we can get this done" spirit.*

Wells

## Forward March

Congratulations! You are taking your first positive steps down the road to getting well. Now it is time to walk farther down the path on your recovery quest.

# Chapter Three

# Getting It Together

*When I was preparing to go to a university hospital outside my home town for surgery in 1992, I thought about the many times I had been asked about my medical history. In the past I had answered as well as I could, but it occurred to me that at different times I might have left things out or guessed the wrong dates.*

*My medical history is complicated, and I wanted to make sure I had everything right this time. I compiled all the information that I thought was important. The computer made it easy to organize it onto a one-page sheet that I took to the hospital with me.*

*Sure enough, I was asked many questions by numerous medical staff the day of the surgery. Each time I pulled out my "medical resume." Without exception, they were impressed and grateful. My sheet was photocopied and attached to the front of my chart.*

*I felt good about having done this, and I think it really helped me participate in my care.*

Mary

## Putting Together Your Medical Resume

The next step toward gaining control is to compile a synopsis of your medical history, a one- or two-page document containing all the information that your healthcare providers should know. Include a recap of any hospitalizations, as well as the year and medical-center location of each incident. Include a list of medications you are currently taking, and any allergies or adverse reactions you have had. Include the names and telephone numbers of any doctors you are currently seeing and a word or two about why they are treating you.

Keep at least one copy of this medical resume on file at home and carry one with you as a handy reference in case of emergencies. Give a copy to every new person who becomes involved in your care. Handing your doctor a complete and up-to-date synopsis of your medical history can save time and it shows that you are actively participating in your treatment.

Pulling all of this information together may seem like too much work, especially if you aren't feeling well. If possible, assign the task to someone who loves details and would appreciate the opportunity to help you.

To make updating easy, enter all of this data into a computer. Ask someone for help if you are unable to do this yourself. A little effort to complete this task up front will save countless hours of repeatedly recalling the same information in the future. It will also ensure that you tell your complete story to each new doctor you visit. Here is a fill-in form for you to follow:

# My Medical Resume

My name _____

My address _____

My phone # (daytime) _____ (evening) _____

My fax # _____

My e-mail address _____

My birthdate _____ My blood type _____

Person to contact in case of emergency:

(Name) _____ (Phone) _____

My insurance provider _____

Policy # _____ Phone # _____

I am allergic to the following (describe reaction):

I am currently taking the following prescription medications (include dosage, frequency and purpose):

I also take the following, either regularly or occasionally (include such things as aspirin, vitamins, herbs, melatonin, etc.):

I have had the following diseases, conditions and medical events:

I have had the following surgeries and/or treatments:

These are the doctors who are currently treating me:

These are the doctors who have treated me in the past:

Other information the doctor should know about me (including special directions for physicians, etc.):

Use only those segments of the form that are relevant to your situation. Adapt them to your own special needs. Later on, you may want to change the format as your condition and/or treatment programs change. Some people create a section on this form called "patient's wishes," to specifically outline which procedures they would (or would not) like performed on them, in case they unexpectedly end up in the hospital. It's your form. Make it work for you. Here are some examples:

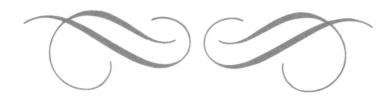

# Medical Resume — Susan Sandeman

**Address:**
123 Main Street,
Charleston, NH 12121

**Birthdate:** 2/15/45

**Telephone numbers:**
123-555-1212
123-555-2121 (fax)

**Emergency contact:**
Robert Smith, 555-1221

**Insurance:**
Cigna PPO
800-555-2221

Group #: 2222
SSN 111-11-1111

**Normal BP:** 90/60

**Blood type:** O+

**Drug allergies (reaction):**
penicillin (hives)
sulfa (rash, breathing difficulty)
codeine (nausea)

Seconal (rash)
Allopurinol (rash)
Darvon (nausea)

**Current medications:**
**Non-Prescription:**
vitamin C, 500 mg.
vitamin E, 400 IU
calcium, 1000 mg.
magnesium 500 mg.
Centrum Silver
Tylenol occasional

**For cardiomyopathy:**
Coumadin 5 mg. daily
Lanoxin .25 mg. daily
Zestril 10 mg. daily

**Doctors:**

| | | | |
|---|---|---|---|
| Primary care | Dr. A | 123-555-6610, | 555-6110 (fax) |
| Oncologist | Dr. B | 123-555-7676, | 555-7766 (fax) |
| Cardiologist | Dr. C | 123-555-7778, | 555-7888 (fax) |
| Gynecologist | Dr. D | 123-555-7878, | 555-7788 (fax) |
| Surgeon | Dr. E | 123-555-8866, | 555-6688 (fax) |

**Diseases, medical events:**
Childhood: chicken pox, measles, rubella
1967    Kidney stones
1982    Large cell lymphoma
        (treated with CHOP therapy and radiation)
1983    Shingles
1992    DCIS, focus of mucinous carcinoma, left breast
1993    Congestive heart failure, cardiomyopathy
        (heart biopsy showed anthracycline cardiotoxicity)
        (treated with above medications)
1995    Mucinous carcinoma of breast, left axilla
        (treated with 9 mos. tamoxifen, oophorectomy)

**Surgeries and hospitalizations:**
1950    Three eye surgeries for strabismus
1953    Tonsillectomy, adenoidectomy
1970    Left oophorectomy, appendectomy
1972    Birth of son Joshua
1975    Birth of daughter Elizabeth
1982    Left axillary lymph node biopsy, New England Hospital
1983    Tubal ligation, New England Hospital
1991    Vocal cord polyp removed, New England Hospital
1992    Left breast biopsy, Boston Clinic
        Bilateral mastectomy, Boston Medical Center
1995    Left axillary dissection, Boston Clinic
        (1/11 lymph nodes positive for mucinous carcinoma)
1995    Right oophorectomy, hysterectomy, New England Hospital

**Medical Record #s:**

| | |
|---|---|
| New England Hospital | 123-555-1000 |
| #07676 | 123-555-1001  (fax) |
| | |
| Boston Clinic | 123-555-1010 |
| #124323 | 123-555-1111  (fax) |
| | |
| Boston Medical Center | 123-555-0101 |
| #046520 | 123-555-1001  (fax) |

# Medical Resume — Jennifer Jones

53 Hill Street
Mill Creek, CA 94444
**Birthdate:** 10/1/55
**CDL#** 99999

**Phone:** 222-555-2121
**Fax:** 222-555-3333
**Blood Type:** O+

**Insurance:**
(primary) Blue Cross
Group# 3333
XDM# 555-22-3333
Phone: 800-888-8288

(secondary) Medicare
555-22-3333
PARTS A & B
Eff. date: 2/1/96

**Contact in Emergency:**

Peter Williams (husband)
222-555-2322

**Drugs:** I am not allergic to any drugs but morphine causes me to hallucinate. Good drugs for me are Zofran (nausea) and Dilaudid (pain).

**Medications:** Daily vitamin pill; Super Cleanse (natural bowel cleanser) 900 mg daily.

**Medical History:** Diagnosis is recurrent mucinous carcinoma with extensive pseudomyxoma peritonei. Origin is either from ovaries or appendix. Problems first arose as ovarian. Have undergone several debulking surgeries (1980, 1984, 1991, 1996, 1996 and two in 1998). Evidence of metastatic disease is apparent. Next treatment (experimental) using heated radio waves to kill tumor is scheduled for 8/10/98.

**Current Condition:** Patient feels okay although energy level is low. Potential for digestive blockage is great.

**Patient's Wishes:** I do not want emergency surgery performed, if at all possible. My goal is *not* to have a total colectomy with ureterostomies performed. In fact, I choose not to have any surgery performed on me unless the prognosis for a satisfactory recovery is possible. If surgical treatment is not possible under these circumstances, then I ask that pain medication be administered, so that I may be made to feel as comfortable as possible.

Signed:_____ Date:_____

**Doctors Currently Treating Me:**

| | |
|---|---|
| (Oncologist) | (Surgeon) |
| Dr. A | Dr. B |
| 12 Webster St. | Hospital Center |
| Mill Creek, CA 94444 | 123 Z Street |
| 222-555-1212 | Mill Creek, CA 94444 |
| | 222-555-1222 |
| | |
| (Internist) | (Gynecologist) |
| Dr. C | Dr. D |
| 32 Center Pkwy. | 123 Z Street |
| Mill Creek, CA 94422 | Mill Creek, CA 94444 |
| 222-555-3322 | 222-555-1234 |

**Other Doctors Who Have Treated Me:**

(Oncologist)                     Dr. E, 444-555-1543
(Surgeon)                        Dr. F, 666-555-1325

**Medical Records At:**

Hospital Center, 123 Z Street, Mill Creek, CA 94444 MR# 1234-7
Stamford Hospital, 333 Serra Street, Stamford, CA 94305 MR# 154-26

**Hospitalization Recap:**

| | |
|---|---|
| 1/21/80 | Removal of 3 ovarian mucinous tumors and 1-1/2 ovaries |
| 10/1/84 | Hernia repair |
| 10/17/84 | Diagnostic laparoscopy |
| 12/3/84 | Hysterectomy and PMP debulking |
| 3/29/91 | PMP debulking |
| 8/30/93 | PMP debulking — removal of 70% of colon and part of the liver |
| 11/14/95 | Complete cytoreduction followed by heated IP chemo, Procedure included removal of cervix, spleen, gall bladder, and remake of diaphragm |
| 11/12/96 | Stage 3 cytoreduction followed by heated IP chemo |
| 4/21/98 | Stage 3 cytoreduction followed by 5 days of IP Taxol |
| 7/1/98 | Stage 3 cytoreduction followed by heated IP chemo |

# Medical Resume — Joan Black

**Address:**      15 Spruce Street, Wilsonville, NV 10101
**Telephone:**   702-555-1111

**Primary Medical Problems:** severe coronary artery disease, degenerative disk disease of the lower spine, TMJ syndrome, ulcers

**Procedures and/or Hospitalizations:**

| | |
|---|---|
| 12/19/97 | Hospitalized w/ chest pain (angiogram by Dr. N) |
| 11/4/97 | Hospitalized w/ chest pain (persantine thallium study showed ischemia) |
| 8/25/97 | Hospitalized w/ rapid heart rate, sweats, nausea, lightheadedness (pacemaker was not working properly) |
| 7/30/97 | Went to ER w/ chest pain (fluid in lungs, high sedimentation rate, pericarditis) |
| 7/12/97 | Hospitalized w/ chest pain (angioplasty of one bypassed vessel that had narrowed, causing slight heart attack (Dr. N) |
| 5/10/97 | Hospitalized w/ unstable angina (Dr. N) |
| 3/19/97 | Hospitalized w/ unstable angina (Dr. N) persantine thallium study showed ischemia problems |
| 12/2/96 | Hospitalized for replacement of pacemaker generator (DDDR Pacesetter Synchrony III generator & atrial lead implanted, Dr. B) |
| 9/24/96 | Hospitalized for angioplasty and placement of OM1 stent (Chicago Heart Institute, Dr. W, became ill while traveling) |
| 5/24/96 | Gastroscopy (Dr. M) found one ulcer and hiatal hernia |
| 4/12/96 | Hospitalized for angioplasty, RCA stent (Dr. N) |
| 4/11/96 | Hospitalized for angioplasty 3 LAD stents (Dr. N) |
| 1994 | Hospitalized for microdiscectomy L4-5 (Dr. T) slight disk bulges still at L3-4 and L5-S1) |
| 1992-96 | Treatment for TMJ syndrome (Dr. L) |
| 1989 | Hospitalized for pacemaker replacement |
| 1979 | Hospitalized for pacemaker implant (for bradycardia) |
| 1975 | Onset of degenerative disk disease of lower spine |
| 1975 | Hospitalized for total hysterectomy (widespread endometriosis) |
| 1974/75 | Hospitalized several times with pulmonary emboli |

**Pacemaker** set at 60 BPM          **Blood Type** O-
**Blood Pressure** generally 140/80

**I am allergic to the following drugs:**
penicillin (hives)
cimetidine (drops white count)
codeine (rash/nausea)

**I am currently taking the following medications:**

| | | | |
|---|---|---|---|
| Procardia XL | 60 mg. | 1x per day | heart |
| Metoprolol | 50 mg. | 1-2x per day | heart |
| aspirin | 5 grains | 1x per day | heart |
| Imdur | 60 mg. | 1-2x per day | angina |
| Nitrolingual spray | 0.4 mg. | as needed | angina |
| Synthroid | 0.05 mg. | 1x per day | slow thyroid |
| Lescol | 20 mg. | 1x per day | cholesterol |
| ibuprofen | 800 mg. | as needed | degenerative disk |
| Carafate | 1.0 gram | w/ibuprofen | ulcer |
| Prilosec | 20 mg. | 1x per day | ulcer |

**My medical insurance is:**
Aetna US Healthcare            ID#: 234-56-7810
P.O. Box 000                   Member Services: 800-756-7039
Fresno, NV 93701               Provider Services: 888-239-1287

**In case of emergency:**        Barbara Jones, 111-555-5115

**These are the doctors who are currently treating me:**
Primary care: Dr. B            Gynecologist: Dr. M
763 Nevada St.                 1 Laurel Lane
Wilsonville, NV 10101          Lakeview, NV 10111
111-555-7000, fax 555-7001     111-555-0100, fax 555-0101

Cardiologist: Dr. N            Neurosurgeon: Dr. T
48 Webster St.                 48 Webster St.
Wilsonville, NV 10101          Wilsonville, NV 10101
phone/fax: 555-7000/555-7001   111-555-6111, fax 555-6112

**These doctors have treated me in the past:**
Dr. C (Surgeon)                111-555-1222
Dr. W (Pulmonologist)          111-555-2121
Dr. S (Gastroenterologist)     111-555-2221

# A Living Will and a Durable Power of Attorney for Healthcare

Even if you choose to indicate your "patient's wishes" on your medical resume, we strongly recommend that you also provide your doctors with one other important document: either a Living Will or a Durable Power of Attorney for Healthcare. Both of these documents protect your interests in case you are unable to make decisions at the time of treatment. Both can be prepared by an attorney, or you can use pre-printed forms available at many drug and stationery stores.

A Living Will specifies the types of treatment you will allow or not allow to be administered to you. Without the information provided by a Living Will, doctors are obligated to provide maximum care and will do everything in their power to prolong your life, even if that is not your wish. Even if family members ask that certain procedures not be performed on you, unless you have given specific written instructions, the doctors will use their best professional judgment, and may prescribe treatment that goes against your family's or your wishes.

A Durable Power of Attorney for Healthcare, the alternative document, allows you to designate your spouse or other loved one to make medical decisions on your behalf if you are unable to do so. Before you give someone else power of attorney for your healthcare, make sure he or she understands your desires with respect to issues like resuscitation, life-support and other important matters.

Keep signed copies of one of these forms with you at all times, and give a copy of it, along with your medical resume, to every doctor who treats you. Update these documents at least once a year and give updated copies to your doctors.

## Organizing It All

At some point, you will recognize the need to "do something" with the masses of papers that start to accumulate. At first it may be easiest to just stick everything into one file folder. Soon, however, you will find that it helps to organize things using some sort of system. This system can be as simple or as complex as suits your personal style. The easiest method is to set up a loose-leaf binder with section tabs and pocket inserts. The first few tabs can be labeled things like "Questions and Answers," "Medical Resume," "Reports," "Literature," and "Resources." As time goes on, you can simply add more tabs and inserts (and binders) as your needs dictate. A little effort on this up front will save you countless hours retrieving this same information again and again in the future.

Some of you may balk at all of this organization stuff. All we can say is, it's a lot easier to disassemble this information afterwards, if you do not like the way that it is compiled, than to try and create organization out of chaos later on down the road.

Putting all of your health-related information, including such things as lab and pathology reports and physicians' notes, into an easy-to-reference system will help you to:

- ensure that you receive better medical care
- put important facts pertinent to your treatment at your fingertips
- be professional and consistent in your communications when dealing with different doctors
- avoid the risk of taking possibly dangerous combinations of medications or engaging in incompatible therapies
- conserve your energy by ending the frantic search for information every time you visit a doctor or go for treatment

By keeping on top of the details surrounding your medical situation, you will feel more in control, be better able to maintain a positive attitude, and be more apt to recognize opportunities which could improve your situation.

# Chapter Four

# How to Get Information

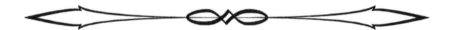

*When I heard that I had cardiomyopathy (a damaged heart muscle), I was stunned and terrified, especially when the cardiologist mentioned a heart transplant. I had originally gone to my internist thinking I might have asthma or a collapsed lung. A heart problem was far from my mind, much less something so final and serious. Even though my emotions were running high, the first thing I wanted was a lot of information. What was the nature of my disease? What course would it take? Should I make specific plans for my life? For my death? What would I have to deal with as the disease progressed? I felt like I was cramming for a college exam — and I hadn't attended any of the classes.*

*I tried to think about where to turn for information. I knew about a local health resource library that a number of friends had used to research their medical conditions. I visited it and proceeded to go through the files that they had, not only about cardiomyopathy, but also on lymphoma and breast cancer (two diseases I had faced earlier). The files contained articles from various sources, including medical journals, books and*

*magazines. I spent quite a few hours over several days reading,*
*photocopying, and searching for information on their computer.*
*Some of the information I found was rather scary, such as the*
*statistics on mortality for patients with dilated cardiomyopathy.*
*But I knew that through all the years that I had confronted*
*previous illnesses, I had never been an ordinary statistic.*
*Actually, reading all the material was somehow comforting,*
*because I learned what I had to deal with. It also helped*
*tremendously as I prepared a list of questions for my next visit*
*with the cardiologist.*

Mary

In this chapter we offer you ideas about how to gather information about your condition. Our list of suggested resources is by no means complete, but it should help you get started. Some of the ideas outlined here will be more practical for you to use than others. Choose those that work best for you. Everyone's needs are different. Some of us want to know all there is to know about our diseases while others are comfortable relying solely on the information our doctors provide. Similarly, the Internet could be the perfect research tool for some, while for others it could be too complicated, expensive (especially if it means going out and buying a computer, modem and telephone line) and confusing. You may prefer going to a library or obtaining information over the telephone.

Depending upon your condition, you may not be able to do a lot of your own research. This is where friends and family can be a big help. Use them!

Think through your goals for obtaining information. Refer to the list of questions that you developed in chapter 2. Use these to focus the nature of your research. Do you want to learn absolutely all that you can about your disease? Or are you first just trying to familiarize yourself with the vocabulary used to explain your disease, its normal course and its treatment options? Or are you interested only in assessing the validity of a specific treatment recommendation?

# Remember: Acquiring Knowledge Takes Time

Too much information, gathered all at once, can be just as useless as no information. Misunderstanding or misinterpreting what you read can occur, especially if the terminology is confusing. For example, many medical terms either sound alike or are spelled similarly but are very different in meaning. Confusing these terms can cause you much unnecessary anguish. Therefore, think about doing your research in "chunks," allowing yourself time to absorb new knowledge in ways that enable you to take the necessary steps without becoming totally overwhelmed by the process.

Here, in no specific order, are some suggested places to search for information.

## Your Doctors' Offices

Ask your doctors how you can learn more about your disease. If they need a little prompting, ask whether they have any educational brochures or videotapes for you to borrow. Be persistent with your questioning. In addition, don't forget that a doctor's office is staffed with a whole team of "behind the scenes" people who may be able to offer you the information that you require.

Although your doctor may not like the idea, also consider starting up casual conversations with other patients in the waiting room about where they found information on their problems. Situations like this tend to bring people together, and although their cases may be different from yours, you may be amazed at the amount of information perfect strangers are willing to share with you. These "brief encounters" can be a really useful resource. Once you get started, however, don't end your search at the doctor's door.

## Other Healthcare Professionals

Nurses, technicians and physicians' assistants are among the most helpful medical professionals. In some cases, they have more practical knowledge than the doctor about how patients with your disease successfully cope with symptoms, side effects and general, day-to-day, ups and downs. Take the time to develop a rapport with them. It will be well worth the effort.

Others who work in healthcare fields, such as research professionals, social workers, health educators and nutritionists, can also be of assistance. In addition, perhaps you have a family friend who is a doctor. Even if this person's specialty is not specific to your disease, he or she might be willing to help you understand some of the medical terminology, point you in the direction of other doctors or medical centers that are known for treating your problem, or simply help you to outline how you can best go about getting assistance.

Even if asking others for help makes you uncomfortable, swallow your pride and ask anyway. If someone declines to help, you are no worse off than before. On the other hand, if they share their knowledge, you will likely be better off.

*I have a wonderful friend who is a physician with lots of contact with other medical professionals and resources. He helps me with research on my various problems. Sometimes I call him when I don't understand the medical terminology in a report. Even though his specialty isn't in the areas of my particular illnesses, he is able to help me gain a useable understanding of what's going on.*

Mary

## Patient Services

Many physician groups, hospitals and HMOs offer an array of patient services, including health educators, nutritionists and social workers. They also have libraries full of books, magazine articles, medical journals and videotapes about many different diseases, procedures and treatment options. These services may be available free of charge, for a nominal fee or on a sliding fee scale. You may still be able to use these services even if they are not a part of your particular medical group. It never hurts to ask. Also, be sure to check with someone in your doctor's office and at your insurance carrier about what patient services are available.

## Health Libraries and Resource Centers

Many hospitals and medical centers have health libraries and resource centers. Some are geared toward the medical community (though still sometimes accessible to the public), while others are specifically geared toward patients, such as the Health Library at the Stanford Shopping Center in Palo Alto, California, and the Planetree Health Library, which is part of the Institute for Health and Healing, located at California Pacific Medical Center in San Francisco. Ask your doctor and friends about what is available in your community and call local hospitals and medical centers to find out what they offer.

Go to one of these libraries or resource centers to find out what is available and how to use the services. Start by looking in textbooks or in medical dictionaries for definitions and descriptions of your condition. Take notes or photocopy pages as you see fit. Later you can read articles from medical journals and magazines. Some resource centers file articles by type of disease or condition. You may also find lists of support groups, research and treatment centers, and physicians who specialize in your disease.

The library or resource center may have access to information via computers, through the Internet or through their own or other subscribable databases. Generally, these computers are set up to be very user-friendly, and someone usually is on hand to help if you get stuck.

Some libraries offer services for a fee that enable you to obtain more extensive research on a specific topic. This can be a big help when you are busy with other things.

Much of the information you find may be quite technical, and there are a variety of approaches to the discussion of medical conditions. It is a good idea to ask someone in the medical field — your doctor, a friend who is a doctor, or another healthcare worker — to help you sort out and understand the information you gather.

# Some Tips for Working with Research Information

- Be sure to note the ***date the work was published.*** Time is an important factor when researching data about your condition. This is not really an issue if all you are trying to find out is a basic description. However, if your goal is to research treatment methods, then the date of your information can be vitally important because treatment protocols can change radically, depending upon the latest scientific research. Make certain in these cases that you are accessing the most up-to-date information possible.
- You may find it helpful to invest in a ***medical dictionary.*** Otherwise, find someone who is familiar with medical terminology to go over the information with you.
- Learn to ***distinguish scientific research*** from anecdotal information.
- When reading about a ***research study or clinical trial,*** note the size and duration of the trial, and when and where it was done. These factors play a part in the value of the research results.
- ***Don't be dismayed by statistics.*** Keep in mind that you are an individual and that you may experience a very different outcome from the published norm. Also, be aware that statistics for a group that is statistically different than you can be very misleading with regard to your situation.
- ***Review your research findings*** with your primary care physician and your consulting doctors.

## Fee-for-Research Services

More and more "fee-for-research" resources are becoming available to patients. You may have read about some of these services in national magazines or your local newspaper. Service fees range from reasonable to very expensive, but for the right person, they can be worth their weight in gold. Rather than conduct your own research, you can hire a company to research the literature pertinent to your condition and compile the information in a manner that makes it easy for you to read and understand. In some cases, they will even meet with you personally to review and discuss the material. Because they are pros at what they do, they usually have access to databases and professional sources that you would not normally come across in your own layman's search. Some also offer a combination of information on conventional medical treatments as well as alternative and adjunctive therapies. As enormously helpful as these resources are, they are not a replacement for your doctor, nor do they constitute a fully considered second opinion.

*The Planetree Health Library* at the Institute for Health and Healing in San Francisco provides personalized literature searches, basic and in-depth health information packets, and information on alternative therapies. The library is dedicated to the principle that access to thorough information empowers patients to make more informed medical decisions. It can be reached at (415) 923-3681.

Two other search services that we are familiar with are Janet Guthrie's *The Health Resource* in Conway, Arkansas at (800) 949-0090 and Gary Schine's web site, *Schine On-Line Services,* at http://www.findcure.com. Gary Schine also can be reached at 800-FIND-CURE. Although both Gary and Janet are cancer survivors, each of their organizations offers research on a wide range of diseases.

Another excellent resource for those with cancer, called *Cancer Care Options,* is in San Rafael, California at (415) 459-0340. The difference between this service and others is that it is staffed by experienced oncologists and research specialists. The treatises prepared by Cancer Care Options deal with specific cancers at various stages of development, providing clients with targeted information about their individual medical situations. In addition, they give patients a kind of decision-making road map to help them evaluate the risks and rewards of various treatments and make the best decisions for themselves.

Here is a list of things you should expect from your fee-for-service researchers:
- They should provide customized information for your specific situation.
- They should be able to cite statistics and results of clinical trials relating to your specific situation.

- If they report on a specific experimental therapy or clinical trial, they should include its eligibility criteria, the results of its preliminary studies, and contact information.
- They should provide you with a list of the databases used in their research.

## Public Libraries

Public libraries have an abundance of books, magazines, tapes and videotapes about health, although only the largest will have the most up-to-date reference materials. Resources vary by size and type of library system, but some or all of the sources listed below will be available to you. It is possible to get facts and even locate books over the telephone, but in all likelihood you will want to visit the library in person to get help finding and using the available sources of information. Library information comes in many forms, including books, magazine articles, directories, dictionaries and other reference sources, newspaper clippings, pamphlets, audio tapes, videotapes, CDs and government documents.

If your illness is a common one, you should be able to find a couple of relevant reference books and perhaps a circulating book or two at your local neighborhood branch. For more unusual needs or more current or in-depth information, you will need to visit a large reference library that contains a range of medical journals covering a number of years. These periodicals will be stored in a number of formats including print, microfiche and microfilm.

Most public libraries have converted their old card catalogs to online resources. Library searches via online indexes are conducted using keywords, which makes the search easier and much more efficient than using the old card catalog system. If you need help with searching, ask a librarian for assistance. A good database to look for is from the Library of Congress, which functions as a national library, making it a good source for works published in the United States. Access to information in magazine articles can also be found online through periodical databases. Many of these include abstracts, so it is easy to determine whether an article will be useful to you without having to read the entire document.

Many public libraries offer Internet access either on site or from home via a modem. Librarians are available to help guide you. In addition, if you locate an article or book through the Internet or elsewhere, your public library can help locate a copy for you. If what you are looking for is not available at your local branch, for a nominal fee you can borrow it through the Interlibrary Loan (ILL) service. Turnaround time varies from a week to several months, depending upon the difficulty of locating the item.

A few libraries are now experimenting with fee-based services to obtain articles and books. For an hourly fee plus delivery, this method can rapidly locate and provide you with requested information. Another document delivery option available through some libraries is FirstSearch, an online database of databases. It is a powerful tool which may have access to more than fifty different databases. For a fee, you can request that a specific article be sent directly to your home or e-mail address.

Stand-alone CD-ROMs are another good source of information. These resources may not be listed in the library's system-wide database, so you need to ask if stand-alone medical CD-ROM databases are available at your library.

Last, but certainly not least, libraries often create their own compendiums of community resources for public use. Such lists or databases are likely to have information about local support groups and other types of helpful services.

## Commercial and Online Bookstores

Bookstores (including medical bookstores and those online such as Amazon.com and barnesandnoble.com) are an excellent source of up-to-date medical information. Many of them encourage you to browse and read selections from the titles they have available. Don't be embarrassed about plopping yourself down in a comfortable chair and looking through what's on sale. In many instances, a book will provide only a paragraph or a chapter of pertinent information. Be sure to bring pencil and paper for note taking when the available information does not justify purchasing an entire book. Most bookstore owners know that if you spend enough time in their stores you are likely to buy something, so they normally encourage you to browse.

If you tell them the title, author and publisher of the book that you are interested in, most bookstores will order any book you want, even if they don't normally carry it. This is especially helpful if you come across a hard-to-find book in the course of your medical research.

## Disease-Specific Organizations and Hotlines

Many organizations focus on particular diseases and disorders. Some of the more well-known ones include the American Cancer Society, the American Heart Association, the AIDS Hotline, the Leukemia Society, the American Diabetes Association, the Arthritis Foundation, the Lupus Foundation of America and the Multiple Sclerosis Society. Some of these organizations are local, and some are national. You will find lists of them in the Yellow Pages or White Pages of your local telephone book or at medical center information offices and health libraries. Many of these organizations have toll-free hotlines. To locate a toll-free number, call 800-555-1212 and ask the operator for assistance.

## Support Groups

Support groups are valuable for many reasons. Apart from the emotional support, there is a real advantage to being able to talk with a group of patients who are all being treated for the same or a similar disease by a variety of doctors from several different medical centers. You can find support groups that meet locally as well as online. They offer a perspective and a wealth of collective knowledge that are hard to find from any other single source. People who participate in support groups also have a willingness to share their experiences with others. Both of us have attended support group sessions off and on in our "health odysseys." In just our first few hours of participation, we each learned more about a variety of treatment programs, clinical trials, and how to deal with side effects than we had in two or three prior months of individual research. We also learned which doctors were preferred by other patients.

To find out about support groups, ask your doctor or your doctor's assistant. Also ask friends, call your local branch of a national disease organization, look for brochures or flyers posted at medical centers and check out those available via your online service and the Internet. You can also call the **Self Help Clearinghouse** at 973-625-9565 for information on support groups in your area. Try to find a group led by someone who not only knows a lot about your type of condition but who also seems "plugged in" to the medical community.

Support groups (like the people who participate in them) all have different "personalities." Some may be a better fit for you than others. Don't be discouraged if you have to try a few out before finding one that suits you. Many groups are focused on patients as they go through specific stages of treatment and healing, while others are targeted to meet the needs of spouses, children and caregivers.

Some support groups charge a nominal fee, or request a donation in exchange for participation. If you are unable to pay, ask the group leader if financial assistance is available.

## Friends and Other Patients

In the same way that support groups can help, friends and other patients with your same type of illness can provide information, at least from their personal perspectives. Even if you never felt particularly close to or had much in common with an individual, take advantage of the knowledge and support that they have to offer. It is amazing how a shared experience like this can bring people together.

*Our friends often ask if we would be willing to talk with a friend of theirs who has been recently diagnosed with a disease like one of ours. We are always willing to share as much infor- mation as we can, and find that there are many other people who feel the same way. Even if we don't have all of the answers that a person needs, at least we can help them figure out a way to find help.*

Mary and Alice

## Health Conferences and Symposiums

Keep your eyes open for information about conferences put on by organizations that focus on your type of condition and the problems related to it. Not only can you learn a lot from the presentations, but you may also benefit tremendously from meeting other people in your same situation. These types of events also enable you to learn about the spectrum of medical services and the latest treatment developments that could be of benefit to you. In addition, they provide you with the opportunity to meet some of the important professionals in the field.

## The Internet and Online Services — Access to Research Data, Articles, Chat Groups, Etc.

*After finding little beneficial information and no hopeful resource to help me fight my cancer, in desperation I started posting messages on the Internet. After about a month of posting weekly messages, I finally started to get responses from doctors, medical researchers and patient "experts." They all suggested that I talk with a surgeon in Washington, D.C., who was pioneering a new treatment procedure. I did. He saved my life in 1995.*

Alice

Access to online services and the Internet offers a wealth of information that was not available to patients just a few years ago. If you decide to conduct research online, do not be surprised to find that you may be more up-to-date on the latest treatment-related information than your doctor. This may especially be the case the farther away you live from large medical research and treatment centers.

Many libraries and medical centers now have computers that patients may use to access the Internet. Some even teach classes on how to go about this. It is also possible to purchase an older model or used computer, modem and printer for a few hundred dollars. New computers fully equipped for Internet use are dropping in price as well. In addition, some of us may soon have access to systems which attach to our televisions and allow access to e-mail and the Internet for a minimal fee.

We have found some excellent books written on this subject. One, entitled *Health Online*, is authored by Dr. Tom Ferguson, medical editor of the *Millennium Whole Earth Catalogue* and a senior associate at the Center for Clinical Computing at Harvard Medical School. Ferguson's book tells people, in plain English, how to access exactly the kinds of information that you will be looking for. He covers all sorts of subjects from corresponding via e-mail, to the use of commercial online services, to signing on to Internet newsgroups, to researching the resources available on the World Wide Web, as well as how to directly access medical databases. In addition, he provides summaries and lists the web addresses of hundreds of health-related information sources. Another very good book that provides information in the same vein is *Your Personal Net Doctor*, published and edited by Michael Wolff.

You should, of course, always look for the most current references when dealing with the Internet as changes to its content occur rapidly.

If you subscribe to a large commercial online service, such as Microsoft Network or America Online, you can easily take advantage of the disease-related health forums and chat groups that they have available. These groups can put you in touch with others who face or have faced your situation. This can be particularly heartening if you have a rare or unusual disorder. Now, via the computer, you can talk with someone thousands of miles away who is going through the same experiences you are. The sharing of information with another in a similar situation can be very comforting. It can also help to save lives, because people are now able to more easily exchange information about successful treatment programs and alternatives.

To subscribe to most any online service, call the company's toll-free telephone number, tell them the kind of computer you have, and they will send you a free sign-up kit in the mail. Once you have registered with a particular service, you can follow their screen directions telling you how to access health-related information.

Internet mail lists (list servers) are another way to access information and meet others with your disease via the computer. Rather than having to go to a newsgroup bulletin board to retrieve messages, you receive those sent via the mail list automatically in your e-mail box. The best of these lists are monitored by a human being, rather than by just a computer program (or mail server), and are governed by a stated list of participation rules. The "Keyword" function available on your online service is a good way to find out about different mail lists.

Other online communication options include Usenet newsgroups (discussion groups). They currently number about 30,000, but lately, many have been overrun with junk mail postings. Anyone can read and reply to messages in Usenet groups, because few are moderated. In our mind this makes them less useful than list servers.

Internet search engines, such as AltaVista, Infoseek, or AOL's NetFind, are also useful in finding disease-specific mail lists as well as the latest research and treatment information. The easiest way to go about this is to type the name of your disease or medical condition into the search box and then press enter. The search engines will locate all information within their scope that contains the term(s) you indicated. You can read through the listed descriptions and go from there directly to the Internet address. One caveat — the ratings that you see attached to Internet addresses are not indicative of the quality of information found therein. Rather, search engines rate addresses by the number of times a word included in your search is mentioned in the web pages.

You can also search through medical documents on the Internet via Gopher. Gophers were in existence before the development of the World Wide Web, and many Gopher sites are now being converted into web sites. Most can be reached by substituting the http:// part of the address with gopher:// followed by the rest of the address. Information found through these sites can be very technical and, at least at first, you may not find them to be the best information resources for you.

As for information regarding specific resource sites, we have listed some of our favorites here, but it is by no means an all-inclusive list. Consider these that we mention as starting points and carry on your own research from there:

- ***MEDLINE*** is a listing of health-related professional articles and their summaries (abstracts). It is available free online and can be accessed through many web pages. Probably the best is through the National Library of Medicine at http://medlineplus.nlm.nih.gov/medlineplus

Many of the Medline sources will allow you to order the full text articles free of charge, while some charge for the service. For a good comparison of offerings by site, check out http://www.medmatrix.org/info/medlinetable.asp.

- *NORD,* which stands for the National Organization for Rare Disorders, Inc., has information on a large number of rare conditions. You can obtain help locating groups specifically focused on a particular disorder through
  http://www.rarediseases.org
  or by phone: 800-999-6673 or 203-746-8958.

- *Doctor's Guide* is a great web site that offers information about the latest research developments affecting treatment of many different diseases. In addition, it provides descriptions of new drugs on the market and links to other recommended medical web sites. The information is updated daily. It is targeted to physicians, so it can get pretty technical. However, it's a great way to keep in step with much of what is happening in the medical field. Address: http://www.docguide.com.

- *Medical Matrix* includes pointers to and rankings of Internet medical resources at
  http://www.medmatrix.org

- *CancerNet* is run by the NCI (National Cancer Institute). This comprehensive site is a must visit for anyone with cancer. It includes gateways to lots of information including listings of current clinical trials, at
  http://cancernet.nci.nih.gov.

- *CanSearch,* another cancer site, is recommended to anyone who wants to search for information about their disease and get the most information in the least amount of time:
  http://www.cansearch.org/canserch/canserch.htm.

- *Findcure* is run by Gary Schine, a survivor of kidney cancer. It is an excellent example of a web site that offers a personal point of view. Gary offers access to a number of cancer-related information resources at
  http://www.findcure.com.

You must evaluate for yourself the benefits of any web site. Here are three questions to consider:

- Is this web site trying to sell me something?
- Is this web site offering me scientific data or personal information?
- Does the information on this site represent expert or personal opinion?

# Chapter Five

# How to Get the Most from Your Doctors

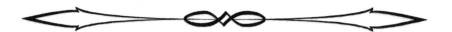

*I used to approach visits to the doctor very differently from the way I do now. I would wait for the doctor to ask me questions, examine me, perform tests, and then tell me what could be done to make me better. While this seemed logical, I often left my appointments feeling frustrated that my questions (which I rarely asked) went unanswered. In addition, I felt that I knew hardly anything about my tests or their results. Bottom line, I wasn't "participating" in my own treatment. Over the years, through trial and error, I have developed a number of techniques that enable me to make more of my doctor visits and help me to feel more in control of my own care.*

Mary

For those in immediate need of specialized medical attention, choosing a physician may be much like going on a blind date. "She's got a great reputation," someone will say. "He's chairman of the department," or "He's the one who treated so-and-so," others will remark. While these phrases may be comforting, they don't offer much substantive information. The chairman of the department may hold that job because he's a better manager than physician. At face value, we simply don't know, but often we make decisions based on "face value" information. We may well have known more about a teenage blind date than we do about the doctors to whom we entrust our lives. And we no doubt spent more time preparing for those dates than we do getting ready for our first appointment with a new doctor.

When you stop to think about it, it's amazing how enthusiastically we leap into a relationship with a physician who we hear is "really good." Often we do this on blind faith, without knowing anything about the doctor. Doctors are not almighty gods. They are human beings with their own character strengths and weaknesses. When we look back on our own experiences, we are thankful that our "leaps of faith" for the most part turned out positive. But for every two of us, there may be two other patients with horror stories about their medical "experiences."

The lesson to be learned is do your homework and use some common sense when building relationships with your doctors.

You are the one best equipped to manage your own well-being. By all means, seek professional expertise and guidance, but remember that no physician can guarantee results in the face of a serious disease. So many factors — physical, emotional, environmental, economic and spiritual — play a vital role. Physicians are important but they can only help you help yourself.

You may be thinking that you already have enough to deal with and you just want someone else to take control of your treatment. Enabling a doctor to direct your medical care is the right thing to do, but don't dump full responsibility for your life onto your doctor's shoulders. It will not help you feel better, and may have the opposite effect by making you feel anxious much of the time and instilling in you a non-productive sense of helplessness.

Getting well is *not* about someone else making you better. As much as others, including your doctor, want to help, it is your life. Take responsibility for it.

## Getting Well Requires a Team Effort

Even the most gifted doctor cannot do her best without your help and input. To get the most out of your doctors' skill and expertise, you must understand how best to work with them — and they, in turn, must learn to work with you. Discuss fundamental issues such as communication and personal philosophy up front, not necessarily in the first minute that you meet, but certainly by the end of your initial appointment. Let your doctor know the issues you want to discuss. Tell him whether you are the type of person who wants to know absolutely every minute detail about your diagnosis and treatment, or whether you feel more comfortable when he is more directive in determining your treatment choices. Be honest in your approach. Don't put on a stoic front if you are quaking in your shoes at the prospect of going into the hospital. Allowing your doctor to see who you really are helps him or her formulate the most suitable treatment plan.

Often there is more than one way to treat a disease. Treatment options involve a variety of factors. Your doctor must understand you in order to confidently recommend the most effective program.

Approaching your doctor honestly fosters a more productive working relationship. If the term "relationship" is uncomfortable for you, then call it a collaboration. Either way, effective treatment depends on clear communication, a solid understanding of mutual strengths and weaknesses, and respect for each other's points of view. Your job is not necessarily to make your doctor feel good about you, but to take full advantage of the skills that he or she has to offer.

*My first visit to an oncologist was disturbing, to say the least. All I kept thinking was, "He's so young." The fact that he had been in practice only one year made me skeptical. Yet he was in a prestigious San Francisco practice. Maybe he'd been first in his class. I was hopeful that he was attuned to the most progressive thought in cancer treatment.*

*I told him I wanted to be a partner with my oncologist and that I also had an appointment with a specialist in Chicago who had spent the past twenty years working with cancer patients and nutrition.*

*"There are a lot of quacks out there," said the oncologist. "If that doctor wants to call me, I'll be happy to speak with him."*

*"What?" I thought. "'If he wants to give you a call...'? You're just out of school. He has worked twenty years to develop a busy, reputable practice and you want him to call you? I don't think so! Strike one. This oncologist is not as open as I would hope or expect."*

*Nevertheless, I proceeded with my questions. Being what some would consider a "health nut," I'd done quite a bit of reading on health and wellness over the past twenty years. It was important to me to be sure my doctor and I were on the same team.*

*Then I asked, "What could I do to strengthen my immune system to be best prepared for the chemotherapy?"*

*"Well," he responded, "one of my patients has taken vitamin E, and another has taken vitamin B, but I really don't think it makes any difference."*

*Strike two. The more I thought about his answers the more angry I became. "If he doesn't know about nutrition," I thought, "at least he could suggest that I walk every day or refer me to the hospital's nutritionist." I left his office and the hospital disappointed.*

*I had to go back to see him the following week to interpret tests he had administered. I thought a lot about what I wanted to say to him the next time we met.*

*When I went for the next appointment, I knew it was important for me to speak frankly. In the examining room, I took a deep breath, looked directly at him, and voiced what had been on my mind. "You can't know what it's like to be in my skin right now. It's scary to be facing cancer without knowing what's ahead. I've done a lot of reading and spoken with other cancer survivors to help me sort through the maze of information. I need to have a heart-to-heart talk with you.*

*"You know, John," — I called him by his first name to help me feel we were on the same level — "after my first visit with you I spoke with a local specialist who has an excellent reputa-*

*tion. When I told him I was going to the Chicago specialist for another opinion, he said, 'I understand he does some very interesting work. If you can send me any information about his treatments, I would really appreciate it.' That, Doctor, is the kind of response I would hope for from my oncologist.*

*"There was one other thing that bothered me during my last appointment with you. When I expressed my interest in strengthening my immune system, I was stunned by your comment that vitamins didn't make any difference. That was a totally unacceptable response for me. I don't expect you to know everything, and I respect what you know, but I come here for direction and support. When a patient comes to you with an obvious interest in being an active partner in getting well, plus an interest in nutrition, you should hear the plea for information. You could have said, 'You know, Barbara, we have an excellent nutritionist here in the hospital. Let me put you in touch with the Community Health Resource Center or with the nutritionist so you can get your needs met.'"*

*The young oncologist listened. He truly heard me. He even shared frankly with me his own impressions of my first visit with him. I told him I appreciated the exchange, and we got on with the reading of my test results.*

*Ultimately, I chose to be treated by another oncologist in the young doctor's practice group. After our exchange, however, he and I respected each other, and my treatment from that office's team of doctors and nurses has been exceptional.*

Barbara

## Help Your Doctor Help You

You go to the doctor because you have a problem that requires medical attention, and your total focus is naturally on yourself. A doctor who takes a dozen or more appointments in a day may face one set of difficult circumstances after another. Add the enormous pressure to hold down costs without compromising the quality of care; the practical difficulty of correlating what may be a baffling array of symptoms to a specific disease and then discerning the proper treatment; and then toss in for good measure any personal problems the doctor is facing in the office or at home, and you have just written a prescription for maximum stress. A physician who specializes in a critical care discipline such as oncology or cardiology may move from one crisis to the next without time to regroup or focus.

You shouldn't have to bear the brunt of the doctor's busy schedule, but don't make matters worse by playing games or being upset when the doctor hasn't memorized your file before arriving in the examination room. By understanding the physician's perspective, you can take steps to help your doctor focus on you and your situation. One important thing you can do is find out what system is used by your doctor's office and then do your best to work within it.

It is only human for a doctor to feel more positive toward patients who take an active role in their own care. Don't push your doctor away by being rude, impatient, uninterested, or close-mouthed about yourself. Even when you don't feel well, strive to be honest, provide feedback, and do your best to understand and support the treatment your doctor prescribes. Be a partner to your doctor in your care. The more you help, the better your doctor will be able to help you.

From our years of experience in and out of doctors' offices and hospitals, we have compiled some practical suggestions for getting the most out of your visits to the doctor. Helping your doctor takes work but is well worth the effort. After all, it is your well-being at stake.

# The Doctor Visit:
## Fifteen Tips You Can *Really* Use

### 1. Before you make your appointment, consider your expectations.

Think of your appointment as an important business meeting and make a list of the things that you need to do to properly prepare. Why do you want to meet with this doctor at this time? What do you expect to get out of this meeting? What do you think the doctor expects of you? How much time will you need for this visit? If you go prepared, you can feel reasonably assured that your appointment will be time well spent.

## 2. Don't expect miracles.

Be realistic. No medical miracles are going to take place during your appointment. Doctor visits are your opportunity to ask questions and to discuss issues and ideas with a knowledgeable source. From your doctor's point of view it is an opportunity to hear from you — to learn your medical history, to understand your concerns, to answer your questions, to discuss your treatment progress and options, and to decide whether more tests need to be administered. If you go with the expectation that something incredible is going to happen, you will be disappointed. But if your preparation is thorough and your expectations are realistic, you will leave your doctor's office feeling good because you have accomplished what you set out to do.

## 3. When you call to make your appointment, be clear about why you want to see the doctor and how much time you will need.

Scheduling nurses cannot read your mind, and they cannot help you if you leave them in the dark. When you call to schedule an appointment, be clear about what you would like to accomplish during your visit.

> *"I would like to see Dr. X about my _____. I was referred by Doctor Y. This will be a first visit for me and I have some questions regarding..."*

Most doctors schedule appointments in ten- or twenty-minute increments. If you will need more time, tell the nurse when you call for the appointment. Don't be afraid to ask about scheduling matters.

> *"How much time does Dr. X usually allow for patient visits? This is my first appointment."*
> *"Some new symptoms have appeared. I have some questions that may take about thirty minutes to get answered."*

Sometimes, requesting the doctor's last appointment of the day will allow you more time to talk without distractions. If this is your first-ever appointment with the doctor, make certain the scheduler knows this. First appointments *will* take more than ten minutes.

If someone else has made the appointment on your behalf, and you did not get a chance to articulate your expectations or time concerns, call the doctor's office prior to your appointment to confirm the appointment and tell them what they need to know.

If you have a fax machine, consider sending a list of concerns, issues or questions ahead of time. This can help the doctor be prepared to make maximum use of the time you spend together.

### 4. Come with information about yourself that will help the doctor.

On your first visit, bring with you a complete but concise medical history. Use the medical resume worksheet in chapter 3 as an example. Make sure to keep this document updated. Give your doctor a copy and keep a folded copy for yourself in your wallet in case of emergency. This will save time for both you and your doctor.

In addition, take time to write a short summary of how you have been feeling, any changes you have experienced recently, and any specific problems you want to address.

If possible, have any ordered tests or procedures completed far enough in advance that your doctor will have the results in time for your visit. If test results were sent to you, bring them to the appointment.

Here is a sample of what one patient prepared before a meeting with her orthopedist:

Patient Name: Sally Gray
Address: 34 Elm Drive          Phone: 555-2711
River City, CA                Fax: 555-2712

Birthdate: 12/25/50           Insurance: Account. #43721
SSN: 123-45-6789

Contact in Emergency: Joe Gray (husband) 510-555-9006

Doctor's Visit — Monday, June 23, 1997
Dr. Q, 1212 Medical Parkway, S. River City, CA,
phone 555-2312

Leg Pain: Pain where the left hip joins with the leg. This began about two months ago. Pain is associated with both jogging and walking. Repetition of either activity brings on the same effect. Pain is dull and constant, although it increases with continued activity (i.e., over a few days it gets much worse). It keeps me awake at night and discourages me from exercising during the day. This is very bad for both my mental and physical health. In order to feel good with cancer, I depend upon keeping moderately active. Depending upon how I feel, I like to walk or slow jog five to six days each week, up to three miles per day.

Foot Pain: I also have extreme pain in my feet (mostly the left foot) when I walk for long distances. This has been a problem for the past year. It does not occur when I wear jogging shoes, only dress shoes (flats or heels). I wear arch supports and this alleviates the problem somewhat. I can sometimes hear and feel a cracking or popping sound, as if the cartilage in my feet is moving in and out of place. With this I get a strange feeling in my toes.

FYI: The top portion of my right thigh is numb. This is a direct result of my last two surgeries. I do have some skin sensation and nerve activity. In fact, the nerves go crazy at times. This keeps me awake at night. The numbness does not interfere with my ability to walk or jog.

Considerations:
· Athletic shoes and orthotics — are they too old?
· I sleep with my left leg pulled up to my chest.
· Egg crate foam mattress pad — is it too soft a sleeping surface?

### 5. Come prepared with questions.

On a sheet of paper, write down your questions and concerns. Leave space after each question, so you can fill in your doctor's response. Also leave space on your sheet for additional questions that come up during the visit. Put asterisks by your most important questions or list them in order of importance.

At the beginning of your appointment, tell your doctor that you have questions, even if you have faxed or mailed them beforehand, so adequate time can be allowed.

Don't leave the doctor's office until at least your most important questions are answered. Don't hesitate to ask the same questions you have asked before — there may be different answers this time. It's also fair to ask your doctor, "What questions *should* I be asking that I'm not?"

If you are preparing for a first visit with a doctor and are not sure what questions to ask, get some help. If you are seeing a specialist, your regular doctor or someone in her office might help you formulate your questions. You can also make an appointment for help from a social worker through the patient resources center at your local hospital, medical center or social service agency. Or you can talk with other people who are experienced in your type of medical situation. This is when contacts from friends or support groups can be very beneficial.

Following is a sample list of questions you might ask:

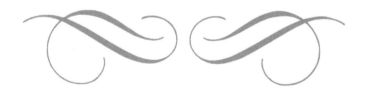

# Questions to Ask My Doctor

1. What is your assessment of my condition at this time?
2. What is my current prognosis?
3. How many other patients with my specific diagnosis have you treated? What were the results?
4. Is there anything that will make a change in my situation? If yes, what is it?
5. What can I do to improve my condition?
6. Are the symptoms I am experiencing normal?
7. Are there specific ways to deal with them?
8. In the long run, what are the potential complications of my condition?
9. What are my chances for recovery?
10. What are the results of any tests I have had?
11. Are more tests in order?
12. If yes, when and what is involved?
13. How will I find out the results of tests?
14. Are there any new studies or test treatments for my condition?
15. If yes, where are these being conducted?
16. Are you in contact with these professionals?
17. What is your plan for my treatment? What are the expected benefits? Are there any alternatives? What are the pros and cons of these?
18. Are there other doctors or health professionals who should be involved in my treatment?
19. What are the short- and long-term effects of the therapy?
20. When should I see you next?
21. How can I get my questions answered between appointments?
22. If I want to get specific information from you, what is the best way to contact you?
    fax? _____ phone message? _____
23. What time of day do you most often return calls?

## 6. Be completely honest.

When your doctor asks you how you are, don't say, "Fine," when you're not. Let all your complaints be known, as silly as they may seem at the time. Now is the time to bring out the sheet that recaps any changes in how you have been feeling. Share this information with the doctor. Sometimes the symptoms you describe are pertinent to your disease, and sometimes they may not have anything to do with your diagnosed condition, but getting your doctor's help in treating them may bring you enormous relief and thus make you feel better overall. Also, be open with your doctor about any apprehensions you have about your diagnosis or its course of treatment. If he prescribes treatment or medication for you and you ignore it, hiding that information will do neither of you any good.

## 7. Bring a tape recorder.

It is very easy to forget what transpires during a visit. So much is happening all at once, that in many instances you are lucky if you remember one-third of what is said during your appointment. Bring a tape recorder and ask your doctor for permission to use it. Taping of sessions is becoming more common, and doctors are getting used to it. Some doctors may feel they are "on stage" and unable to be as frank, but other doctors even provide tapes and recorders for their patients to borrow during appointments.

## 8. Bring a friend.

It helps to have an extra set of ears and someone taking notes during your visit. Ask a friend, spouse or other family member to accompany you. You can discuss your visit afterward to make sure you thoroughly understand what the doctor said. Of course, two people hearing the same conversation may come away with different understandings of what was communicated.

These differences in understanding can be productive, however, if dealt with in the right way. Maintain an open mind if your appointment partner comes away with a different perspective than you do. Talk it out. If necessary, call your doctor or someone in his office for further clarification. However, if your differences in understanding or opinions about how to proceed are too great and cause excessive stress, ask someone else to accompany you the next time.

> *I am shy by nature, so I find it very difficult to talk with my doctors, but I now have an e-mail relationship with the clinical research coordinator for one of my oncologists. Because I am in a clinical trial, she needs to contact me every week. At first she would phone me, but often it was hard to make contact. Now we use e-mail and it works great. I ask her all my questions and she sits in on my visits with the oncologist and often helps me get the answers to my questions. It is not an ordinary way of doing things, but it works for me.*
>
> Pam

## 9. Be sure to receive clear explanations of any tests, procedures, and medications.

If your doctor wants to order tests, procedures or new medications, ask why they are indicated, whether they are necessary, and what they should accomplish. Ask how and when results will be evaluated, and ask about possible alternatives.

Always ask your doctor about the desired effects and any possible side effects. Whenever possible, talk with others such as nurses, lab technicians, pharmacists or others familiar with the procedure or medication. Understand the implications before you agree to anything. As a patient you need to be fully aware that whatever action you take may end up having a negative effect. This doesn't mean that you shouldn't undergo the test or take the medication, but a realistic understanding of what is involved will go a long way in helping you to deal successfully with the consequences. We go into more depth about these situations in chapters 9 and 11.

## 10. If there is a decision to be made, ask your doctor what he would do if you were a member of his family.

You will need to make your own decisions based on many factors, including calculated odds, your own desires, and those of the people around you. Keep in mind that many of the decisions you make are personal and not medical, although medicine may be involved. Still, it can be helpful to know what your doctor would do in your shoes. Some doctors may not like it when you ask this question, but most will respond honestly.

Sometimes your doctor may come to your appointment with a specific set of recommendations that you do not feel comfortable with. In this case, explain your hesitation and need for alternatives so the doctor can understand your point of view. You can learn a lot about your doctor by watching and listening to how he responds to you.

### 11. Repeat back to the doctor what you have heard.

When we hear upsetting news we tend to react with denial, and may block out what is being said. Therefore, say to your doctor, "I would like to understand correctly what you said..." and then state in your own words what you believe he said. This may seem unnecessary or even embarrassing at first, but it can be very helpful by allowing the doctor to immediately correct any misunderstandings, which may later save both of you a lot of time and energy correcting mistaken impressions.

### 12. Keep your own record in your own words of your medical visits.

After your appointment, take a couple of minutes to jot down what you learned and accomplished from your visit. You can do this in a log format. Some patients even keep a separate notebook for each doctor and record their thoughts after every visit. Compare these notes with your written expectations, to make certain that you are on track and are doing your best to get your needs met.

### 13. Have the doctor send you a written report of the visit, and ask him to copy it for others actively involved with your case.

Encourage your doctor to give you written feedback. It will give you and others who are treating you a good understanding and record of your meeting, and will give you a chance to check for and immediately correct any mistakes. You, as the patient, are the best proofreader for your own record, because you know more details about yourself than anyone else does.

**14. Find out how to get your questions answered between visits.**

Often, you may have questions that do not require another full appointment with your physician. Ask your doctor how best to get these needs addressed.

Some doctors take messages through their receptionists or voice mail and then return calls at a specified time of day. If so, find out when that time is so you can be available. Others ask that questions be directed to a nurse, nurse manager, physician's assistant, or someone else in the office, who will then provide you with the answer or refer it to the doctor. Whatever the system, find out how it works and plug into it. Be as specific as you can when stating your questions, so that the answers provided will be useful to you. Also, be nice when you approach members of the doctor's staff. Show your appreciation for their efforts on your behalf. You will catch more flies with honey than with vinegar.

If you have a fax machine, ask the doctor for permission to fax your questions. He or someone else in the office can then answer them at a convenient time and fax the responses back to you. This method works especially well when you want to receive test results between appointments.

**15. Let your doctor know if improvements need to be made to the office.**

Part of your relationship with your doctor is the service and support offered by his staff, including nurses and administrative personnel. If any of these people fail to respond satisfactorily to your requests, tell the doctor. Many doctors are unaware when they are not being well-served by staff.

## A Doctor's Point of View

Although the focus of this book is the patient's viewpoint, we thought you might be interested in what a doctor has to say. Here is one perspective.

*It has been my good fortune to enjoy thirty years of medical practice, during which I have had the privilege of working with many fine men and women, doctors and patients alike.*

*Much is made today of doctors who are incompetent or who do not act in what they understand to be their patients' best interests. I know this happens, but certainly not to the extent that some would have us believe. Patients who enter into a relationship with a doctor aiming to find fault with the treatment that is delivered do themselves and the medical profession a great disservice. Your doctor is not your adversary. If you believe he or she is, then get a new one.*

*Each patient is, indeed, unique. On the other hand, part of Western medical science is dependent on classifying. Doctors need to do some classifying in order to bring their experience to bear to help patients.*

*A doctor's advice cannot be off the top of his or her head. The medical community has strict requirements for diagnosis and treatment, which a physician ignores at his or her peril. Sometimes it may seem that time and money are wasted in pursuit of these requirements; patients have the right to refuse tests and treatments, but they must be offered.*

*In addition, just as patients are trying to understand doctors, so are doctors trying to understand patients. Patients need to contribute to doctors' knowledge and understanding of them. The relationship is a most complex one. Not only are physicians trying to analyze patients from the standpoint of arriving at a diagnosis and recommended plan for treatment, but also to ascertain the many personality and social factors that will affect any course of action.*

*Doctors want to help you achieve the best results within the realm of what they know to be possible. They go for "cures," and may look less at things like expense and diminished quality of life than you do. Therefore, they not only want, but in fact they need you to listen to the likely outcomes expected for various treatments and choose what you think will be best for you. The key to success in this is frankness and a willingness to trust on the part of both parties. Of course, some tact is also required.*

*Taking steps to educate yourself can be positive, but keep in mind that it took your doctor years of training and experience to get where he or she is. Have some respect for the skills that he or she brings to your situation. There are still some doctors whose confidence in their treatment is so strong they will not negotiate with you. Some of the best practitioners I have known fit this description. It all comes down to a matter of personal choice. If you know that the physician is skilled and you are willing to submit, you may be very well served.*

*Most physicians are anxious for you to fully understand your disease, its treatment possibilities and its prognosis. If you do not understand all of these, keep asking for answers until you do.*

Dr. C

## If You Are Having Problems with Your Doctor

Like any other relationship, not every collaboration with a doctor works out. Sometimes, no matter how good a doctor's reputation, or how much we want that doctor involved in our care, the combination of personalities or communication styles just isn't healthy. Usually problems arise from attitudes or an inability to relate well together. If you are having problems working with your doctor, the best course may be to part company.

Before you decide to end the relationship, however, try to talk to your doctor about your problems. If this is too difficult to do in person, write a letter. Be honest, but tactful. Your honesty may result in a positive dialogue that will resolve most of your difficulties.

Ask your doctor how to improve your communication, or talk with someone on his staff for advice and feedback. If the relationship is truly not working out, your doctor and those in his office probably realize it too.

If you are uncomfortable approaching someone in the office, talk with your primary care physician or with a social worker or patient advocate at your local hospital or medical center.

Ask yourself, honestly, whether you are contributing to the problem. If so, consider whether or not you can — or want to — alter your behavior.

If, after all this, you believe that you and your doctor will never be able to come to terms, then it is time for a change. As difficult as this action is, it is a right step in gaining control of your health. Do not hesitate to take action because you are worried about hurting your doctor's feelings. Your own best interest is most important. Be sure, however, that you have someone else to go to who is competent and available.

There are many ways to "fire" your doctor, but the best way is with respect and dignity. Keep in mind how you would feel if you were on the receiving end. Now is not the time to burn any bridges. Your message can be communicated gently and professionally in person or through a letter, such as one of the samples outlined on the following pages.

If you believe in the type of treatment offered by your doctor, but cannot work with his or her personality, you may want to consider asking for a recommendation or a referral to another doctor. If you truly respect the doctor's medical capabilities, this approach allows a way for him to remain part of your care on a consulting basis. If you are feeling the pain of your relationship, chances are your doctor feels it too. He may welcome the opportunity to end a difficult relationship by recommending another doctor whose bedside manner might better match your personality.

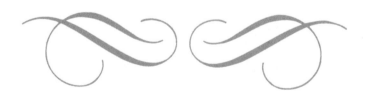

## Sample Letter for Changing Doctors Within the Same Medical Practice

*Dear Dr. _____:*

*Thank you for (meeting with me...). I appreciate your taking the time to help me understand my diagnosis and outline my options for treatment. After much thought, however, I have decided that I need to make some changes regarding my medical care. While I sincerely respect you and appreciate the care you have given me, I feel the need to see someone else (i.e., with a less hectic schedule, or with whom I feel more comfortable). I would like to stay within your medical group, however, because it is one of the best, and I hope you will feel comfortable referring me to one of your colleagues. Again, I am grateful to you for the care you have given me, and I trust that you understand my reasons for this change.*

*With gratitude and appreciation,*

_____

*Signed*                          *Date*

## Sample Letter for Changing to a Doctor Outside the Medical Practice

*Dear Dr. _____:*

*This letter may be as difficult for you to read as it is for me to write, and for that I apologize. After much thought on the subject, I feel that I must make a change regarding my medical care. While I respect your abilities, it has become clear to me that we do not work well together. Therefore, my plan is to seek medical assistance elsewhere.*

*I would like to pick up my medical records at a mutually convenient time. I will contact your office to arrange this.*

*I am grateful for the care you have given me and I hope you understand my reasons for this change. Thank you for all of your help and best wishes to you and your staff.*

*With appreciation,*

_____

*Signed*                            *Date*

# Chapter Six

# When and How to Get Another Opinion

*Following my surgery for a routine hysterectomy, I waited for my doctor to call me with a pathology report. Nearly two weeks went by and still he had not telephoned, so finally I called him. He told me that the supposedly benign cyst he had removed was not benign after all, but malignant. He also told me I should not be overly concerned because he had consulted with two gynecological oncologists and they said that most patients did not have problems after my type of ovarian cancer had been removed.*

*I hung up the phone in a state of utter shock. I could not remember the name of the type of cancer he mentioned or the name of the pathologist who made the diagnosis. All I could remember was the word — cancer. I am an intelligent, well-educated professional who has spent her entire life in medical research, and I still turned to jelly when I heard the word cancer. I was frightened and, in spite of my professional experience, knew nothing about the problem he had described. After allowing myself a few minutes to calm down and stop shaking, I called the doctor back. This time I wrote down the name of the condition and the name of the pathologist. Then I called my husband so that I did not have to face the rest of that day alone.*

*Instead of eliminating my earlier symptoms, the surgery only seemed to make things worse. While my doctor was continuing to assure me that all was well, I was in increasing pain and rapidly losing weight. Little did I know at that point that my trip through the medical maze was just beginning. Further study and many opinions later revealed that I did not have ovarian cancer, but colon cancer in which the primary tumor originated from the appendix. The ovarian complication was actually a metastasis, which ruptured and spewed mucin into my abdomen.*

Pam

## Reasons to Look for Other Opinions

Undergoing treatment for a life-threatening disease is no "small deal." It often involves huge personal risks, major changes in your lifestyle, and a big commitment of time and money. Given this reality, it is a good idea to get as much input as possible before launching into any treatment program.

Obtaining more than one opinion about your diagnosis or your treatment options is usually a good idea. The process, however, requires energy, planning, organization, and an understanding of accepted procedures. Some people are reluctant to make the effort. It's up to you, but opening your eyes to other opinions can maximize your chances for improved health and put you psychologically more at ease.

## When to Consider Another Opinion

Think about obtaining a second opinion in these circumstances:
- when you are attempting to establish or review a diagnosis
- when you must make treatment decisions
- when you are thinking about changing the course of your current treatment

- when you are trying to decide whether or not to stop treatment or considering what your next steps should be
- when you become uncomfortable with your doctor

## Second Opinions Regarding Diagnosis

Any diagnosis of a life-threatening disease is hard to take, but sometimes you have valid reasons for not wanting to believe what you've been told. It may just be a feeling or your doubts may arise as the result of your research. Either way, if you are not convinced the diagnosis is correct, you may want to look for another opinion.

The evidence leading to a particular diagnosis may be based on clues (symptoms) that are not always black and white. Scientific analysis of test results might suggest a certain conclusion, but unless your case is a clear-cut, textbook example of your disease, the symptoms could also indicate something entirely different. Your doctor almost always works with less information than she would prefer.

Even when scientific procedures are used, the interpretation of the results may be more art than science. Two or more pathologists looking at your tissue specimens may reach entirely different conclusions. Furthermore, the tests used to determine a diagnosis may vary in type, quality and outcome based on several factors including the lab and the equipment used for the evaluation. Also, no matter how careful or competent a lab technician is, everyone can make a mistake. As a result, sometimes test reports are incomplete, inconclusive, or based on faulty input.

Whatever the reason, if you have any question about the accuracy of your diagnosis, get a second opinion. At the very least, you will confirm the original diagnosis and be prepared to move ahead with your treatment plan.

*I was diagnosed at one medical center as having breast cancer. After surgery, based upon my surgical pathology report, I started a five-year course of hormonal therapy recommended by my oncologist and the hospital tumor board. A few months later, a genetic counselor looked at the report and expressed concern that it did not contain enough information. She said it was more like a "sketch, rather than a completed oil painting." She referred me to a world-renowned breast cancer pathologist at another medical center to get a second opinion. He discovered an error on the original report. As a result, I went back to my medical center, where my case was re-reviewed and the second diagnosis was confirmed. As a result of the new diagnosis, tumor boards from both medical centers recommended a different, more aggressive treatment. Based on this new information, my doctor completely changed my treatment protocol. I am convinced that the second opinion helped save my life.*

Elisa

## Second Opinions to Explore and Review Treatment Options

Even when you and your doctors agree on your diagnosis, and even if you are comfortable with the recommended treatment protocol, we believe you should consider second opinions in order to fully explore the treatment options that are available to you.

In most cases, your doctor will present only one or two choices for treatment. Using his best professional judgment, based upon his own research and experience, he will describe what he believes is the best course for you to follow, which is usually the one he feels most comfortable administering. His recommendation, however, may or may not be the best choice for you. *Only you can make that decision and then only after you have adequate information about the full range of available options.*

When you are buying a house or a new car, do you buy the first one you see or do you shop around? Deciding how to treat a serious illness is at least as important as buying a house or car. You may ultimately choose your doctor's original recommendation, but the important thing is to make the decision that is best for you after considering as many factors as you can.

## Second Opinions as Confirmation

Another reason for a second opinion is to confirm the treatment you have chosen. It can build your confidence to know that other experts agree with the diagnosis and treatment plan you are following. In addition, outside experts may be able to clarify aspects of your disease or its treatment that your own doctors were unaware of or were not able to explain clearly to you. This may be particularly important when your local hospital does not specialize in the treatment of your condition. However, the local facility may be able to administer your treatment under the guidance of others who are up to date on the latest developments.

## Choosing the Best from an Imperfect Set of Options

Unfortunately, when dealing with disease, you may be forced to choose from a less than ideal set of options. Deciding which option to follow is not easy and you may need to select a treatment program based upon a combination of good and not-so-good choices. For example, you may prefer Dr. A, but if his practice is located in another city, you may not want to travel to receive treatment. Or, a certain treatment may offer you the best chance for success, but its side effects are devastating.

By exploring your options, you will have the opportunity to seek the best the medical community has to offer, and you may also be able to tailor a program that includes positive aspects of several alternatives. Say, for example, that Dr. X, who lives in another state, has developed a protocol that shows promising results in the treatment of your disease. It may be possible to work out an arrangement whereby your hometown doctor is able to administer the treatment under the supervision of Dr. X. This option offers you the comfort of being able to stay home yet still enables you to take advantage of the newest medical thinking.

Creative solutions may not work out in every case, but you will never know unless you ask.

# Six Factors to Consider When Determining Your Treatment Program

1. What are my treatment *options?* (These include receiving no treatment.)
2. In what different *ways* can I receive my treatment?
3. Is it *geographically* important where I receive my treatment?
4. How *long* must I be in treatment? What choices do I have with regard to this issue?
5. What *lifestyle factors* are important to me as I undergo treatment?
6. What *possible aftereffects of treatment* should I be aware of, both short- and long-term?

The rest of this chapter is devoted to guidelines and suggestions about how to make the process of obtaining a second opinion easier. Keep in mind that second opinions can be appropriate at every stage of your diagnosis and treatment.

## Things to Consider When Seeking Other Opinions

Before you decide to look for other opinions, here are some things to be aware of:

**The process requires energy.**
You may feel exhausted, ill or overwhelmed emotionally and are unable to take on one more thing. This is where the support of others is so important to help you with the process.

**The process takes time.**
Extra time may be a luxury you feel you do not have. Doctors sometimes put pressure on patients to start treatment immediately after diagnosis or surgery. Don't let anyone rush you into a situation where you feel uncomfortable, no matter how critically ill you are. You need

to allow yourself adequate time to get comfortable with your treatment decisions. If you don't, it will be harder for you to muster the personal strength you need to help your doctor fight your disease. Taking a few days to sort out your thoughts is usually not going to make the difference between life and death. If your doctor puts pressure on you to start treatment right away, ask him if you are genuinely risking your life by postponing treatment for a couple of weeks. Chances are, the answer will be no.

**The process can cause stress.**

You (and your physician) may feel that seeking other opinions calls your doctor's credibility into question, which can cause stress. But if your doctor responds negatively because you want to explore other options, you may gain an important insight into his personality — and reconsider whether he is the right person to be directing your care.

**Seeking other opinions involves making difficult decisions about which protocol and which doctor to choose.**

If you consult with doctors from three different medical centers, you will likely receive at least two different treatment recommendations. This is more likely to be the case if these centers are located in different geographic areas. These differences of opinion put you in the difficult position of having to choose what to do, even though you have no experience or knowledge to help you.

In addition, choosing one treatment protocol may cut off your options regarding future treatment possibilities. Therefore, if you are interested in pursuing a particular therapy, find out how the treatment will impact other options you may want to consider in the future.

**Financial factors may be an issue.**

Your insurance may not cover the cost of obtaining a second opinion. On the other hand, some insurance companies require second opinions. In other cases, your insurance may cover second opinions only if they are sought from "participating providers" — that is, doctors who are pre-authorized by your insurance carrier. Regardless, most insurers will not reimburse you for travel costs associated with a second opinion.

Although important, these considerations are obstacles that are well worth overcoming if they stand in the way of the best solution to your medical problem. Keep in mind that getting another opinion may actually save your life.

# How to Find Out Where to Go for Other Opinions

**Ask your primary care physician.**

He may have referred you to the specialist who gave you your original diagnosis and treatment plan, but he may also recommend other specialists as well.

**Ask friends and fellow patients.**

Seek out those with similar conditions. Support groups can be very helpful for these kinds of referrals.

**Ask a physician who works for a research service or organization.**

These doctors are often aware of the latest developments in treatment protocols.

**Contact other medical centers.**

Ask whether or not they offer formalized second opinion services. Also ask for the names of affiliated doctors who specialize in your disease.

**Call hotlines such as 1-800-4-CANCER.**

Many hotlines are listed in the white pages of the phone book under disease categories.

**Check for information at health resource centers, hospital libraries, bookstores, or your public library.**

When looking through these reference materials, try to identify those medical centers that have a broadly recognized reputation for treating your specific disease or condition.

**Check the Internet for name of specialists and treatment centers.**

Subscribe to mailing lists that focus on your disease and ask for recommendations from other subscribers. Note the names of doctors (and their affiliated medical centers) who direct or author pertinent research that you come across when searching medical databases.

**Ask other medical professionals.**

Nurses, researchers, lab and other technical professionals may be able to offer referrals.

**Look beyond your geographical area.**

If you are serious about exploring a wide range of options, you will probably have to solicit second opinions from experts outside of your local area. Treatment programs within specific areas tend to be similar. Therefore, if you live in California, check with experts on the East Coast, in the South or in the Northwest. Also, don't be afraid to look to Europe, Asia and beyond, especially if you have a rare condition. Be aware, however, that the farther afield you go, the harder it may be for you to check the medical credentials of so-called experts.

## Four Steps to Use When Getting Other Opinions

**1. Call to request an appointment once you have determined where you want to go.**

Be sure to find out the name of the contact person in the office and how to reach him or her (phone, fax, address). Obtaining second opinions is a relatively common practice these days, so do not be shy about making the calls. When you call be sure to confirm that the doctor offers second opinions and that she will see you with that proviso.

Sometimes, when a physical examination will not provide the consulting doctor any more relevant information, it is possible to obtain a second opinion without having to be present. Often, test results or X-rays can be forwarded to the second doctor for review and interpretation.

Don't forget to find out everything the second opinion doctor will require for your consultation. This will probably include copies of all recent scans, X-rays, pathology slides, blood samples and their accompanying reports, as well as your medical records and notes from your doctor. Here is where your record keeping and preparation can really pay off.

## 2. Draw up a "consultation worksheet."

List all of the details you need to keep track of in pursuing your second opinions. Information should include the names, addresses and phone numbers of all your prospective second opinion providers. Also include a checklist of pertinent records you will need copies of, along with where they are located (address, phone/fax numbers, contact name) and your medical center identification number. A sample worksheet is outlined on the following page:

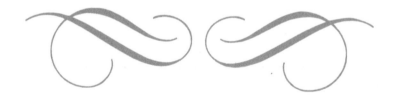

# Consultation Worksheet

Pathology slides
Write a brief description of the content of each set of slides as well the date that they were prepared and the location and phone number where they are stored.

Original X-ray films and scans
Write a brief description outlining the portion(s) of the body captured by each set of X-rays as well as the date of each procedure and the location and phone number where the originals are stored.

Summaries
These include discharge summaries, copies of your medical histories and physicals, as well as lab reports, X-ray reports and treatment records. Note a description of each summary, the date that it was prepared, and the location and phone number where it is filed.

List of locations where medical records are stored
Include a notation of each medical record number and the location and phone number where each is stored.

List of doctors you are seeing as consultants
Include each doctor's phone/fax numbers, address, and the name of your contact person in each office.

List of doctors and medical centers involved in your care
Include each doctor's phone/fax numbers, address, and the name of your contact person in each office.

**3. Gather together all of your pertinent records and information as requested by your consulting doctors.**

This can be quite a burdensome task, and many patients, having done it once, make it a point to keep their own copies of as much information as possible, so that they are prepared for the next time they need to seek a second opinion. Always keep your "at home" files up to date with reports of new tests and doctor visits.

Allow adequate time to gather these materials. If the consulting doctor requests X-rays, slides or other materials, you will have to allow a few days for the information to be gathered. You may also have to sign a release accepting responsibility for these materials. If possible, pick up your records yourself or have someone pick them up for you. This could shave a couple of days off the process.

Unless specifically requested to do so, do not send your records ahead if you are personally meeting with your second opinion doctor. Instead, carry them with you and give them to the person who checks you in. Records can too easily be lost or misplaced if they are mailed. If you must mail materials, call to ascertain that they arrived. If your records have not arrived by several days before your appointment, consider rescheduling it.

Sometimes your specialist or primary care physician will help you with this materials-gathering process or act as an intermediary for the receipt of slides and scans, but more often than not, you will have to assume total responsibility for it.

> *I had hoped that my primary care physician would orchestrate the whole process of getting other opinions. He was supportive of the process, but in the end I had to set up all the appointments and accumulate the records. I did get his help with having records sent to his office, and I got his advice about the protocol and practical procedures.*
>
> Mary

Laws pertaining to your right to access your medical records vary by state. Our advice is to proceed with your request on the assumption that you have a right. If your request is denied, ask why and under what terms you are able to obtain access. In some cases you may have to engage the help of an attorney or consumer action group. See chapter 9 for more detailed information on how to obtain your medical records.

## 4. Follow the guidelines from chapter 5 regarding doctor visits.

Meeting with your second opinion doctor is an especially important occasion. Invite someone to accompany you and come prepared with questions and a tape recorder. Take time to prepare for your meeting. Write out, either in paragraph or bullet-point form, what your present doctor has told you about your diagnosis, prognosis and treatment recommendations. Give this to the second opinion expert, or use it as a reference for "talking points" during your visit.

## Questions to Ask Second Opinion Doctors

Include the following among your questions for your second opinion doctors:

- Do they have any differences of opinion regarding any aspect of my case?
- Is the treatment they suggest the same as those generally given to others with my same condition, or is it designed with my particular situation in mind? Does my situation warrant consideration of any changes in the routine strategy?
- What is the likely outcome if I do not opt to follow this course of treatment?
- Will this treatment possibly require me to alter all or some of my normal daily activities? If so, in what ways?
- Once I finish this treatment, how frequently should I return for check-ups? What types of tests should I have done and how frequently should I have them?
- Are they willing to participate in my care, either as primary treatment doctors or as consultants?

The consulting doctor should tell you in understandable language how much benefit a given treatment will provide you and how well the evidence supports this expectation. He should also explain any risks or possible adverse effects, both short- and long-term. When you receive conflicting opinions, be sure to ask each doctor what the basis for the controversy is.

Ask your consulting doctors to send copies of their reports to you and your primary physician, as well as to anyone else important to your case. Keep your own records, including your thoughts on what you think each doctor said. Then compare these journaled thoughts with the reports the doctors send summarizing your visits. You may even want to send your notes to your consulting doctor for review.

## How to Evaluate Treatment Recommendations

Once you have accumulated these treatment recommendations, how do you make decisions based on the information gathered? Go about it the same way you would objectively make any other important decision.

First, outline in writing what is involved in undertaking each proposed protocol. List in two columns the positive and negative aspects of each program. Following is a sample grid to help you visualize what we mean:

## Second Opinion Matrix

| Doctor | Diagnosis/ Prognosis | Treatment Plan | Pluses | Minuses |
|--------|----------------------|----------------|--------|---------|
| Dr. A  |                      |                |        |         |
| Dr. B  |                      |                |        |         |
| Dr. C  |                      |                |        |         |

There is no right or wrong way to do this. You can make the evaluation process as simple or as complex as you like in order to determine which protocol will be best suited to your needs and temperament. Consider assigning numerical values to your lists of pluses and minuses in order to ascertain which plan offers you the most palatable mix of options. Use the tools you feel comfortable with to make your determination. Here are some considerations to think about as you get started with the evaluation process:

- What are the calculated five- and ten-year survival rates for the protocols being considered?
- How will each of the protocols affect your life in the short and long term? Will your desired treatment require that you travel long distances and spend extended periods of time away from home? If so, how do you feel about that? Will you have an adequate support system in this "away" location to help you get through your treatment?
- If you choose an out of town location for treatment, how will you handle follow-ups?
- How do the different treatment protocols fit your own approach to life? Are you a risk-taker, or do you prefer to live life in a more conservative manner? For example, if one treatment is riskier than others but possibly offers a slightly better chance for remission, how do you feel about this option?
- How do you feel about the doctors involved with each of the treatment protocols? Do you feel more comfortable with any one of them?
- What are your insurance considerations? Will your carrier cover the costs associated with any of these therapies, or will you be limited in what you can choose?
- Are you able to combine any of the options to better suit your needs? Be creative in thinking about the possibilities.

If you are having a hard time coming to a decision, make an appointment with a trusted physician to talk things over. You might also consider asking your doctor to present your case at a multidisciplinary or specialty case conference, so that a group of doctors can discuss your case and offer you their collective advice.

## After You Have Made Your Decision

Once you have made your decision, make copies of all paperwork for your files and return the originals of everything to their original sources.

Communicate your decision to the doctors involved. Let them know the course you intend to take and under whose care. If you would like to remain in contact with any of these doctors for future consultations, let them know that, too.

Be positive about your prospects and proud of the fact that you have taken charge of the process. Be confident, knowing you have fully explored your options and selected the path that is best for you.

# Chapter Seven

# Putting Your Wellness Team Together

*As I learned to deal with my cancer, I found that the tools that were most helpful to me were a very nurturing husband with a good sense of humor, a friend (also a breast cancer survivor) who provided me with good referrals, and a support group whose collective knowledge and acceptance enabled me to carry on.*

Mary Frances

It takes great effort to cope with a serious or life-altering illness. Because you are in a fight for your life, you need a lot of help from others to successfully manage your situation. Under normal circumstances we rarely stop to think about how much we depend on the help and cooperation of others. But when you have a life-altering disease, having a high level of dependable support can make all the difference in how well you feel.

# Whom to Confide In

Some people choose to deal with their illness by not confiding in anyone, at least at first. Privacy is an important issue, and the notion that others will be aware of one's most intimate problems can be unsettling. Others can't wait to spread the news, either out of relief that they finally have a name for their situation or in hopes that others will respond to them in a supportive fashion. Neither route is perfect. Whichever way you choose to go, recognize that there are bound be some bumps and surprises along the way. Here are some things to think about before confiding in others.

## What is your motivation in telling others?

Why do you believe others need to know about your diagnosis? What do you expect to get out of sharing your information? Perhaps most importantly, are you prepared for the possibility that their reaction may not be what you anticipate? Many times we are eager to share information about ourselves in the hopes it will bring us closer to those whom we like or love. Unfortunately, this does not always happen. Your sharing may cause others to shy away, either because they do not have the same interest in further developing the relationship, or because they simply don't know how to respond. Be clear about your motives and try to be sensitive to the feelings of those around you, even though you are the one in crisis. A little discretion will save you from having to nurse hurt feelings in addition to everything else.

## What and how much do others need to know?

This is an important question because your actions today may affect your future. If you are employed, does your illness affect your job performance? Does your employer have a right or need to know? Will your illness change your appearance or emotional behavior? There are laws in place to protect you from discrimination, but do you really want to have to go that far to protect yourself? Even if your employers and coworkers don't openly change their attitude toward you, will disclosure affect your prospects for future promotions or other opportunities? Our belief is that you *should* share information about your situation with those few people at work who really need to know, but not necessarily with all your coworkers.

## What are the positive aspects of telling others?

Having said all of the above, there are some very positive aspects of sharing your personal information, especially with those closest to you. First of all, you are likely to receive needed emotional, physical and perhaps even financial support. Others may be more forthcoming in their offers of assistance if you are open regarding your needs. In addition, the more people who know about your situation the greater the possibility that someone may be able to provide you with a referral to a doctor or suggest some good ideas. Talking about your disease may also help you work through emotional issues you are wrestling with and thereby help you feel better faster. Being open with others about your situation, however, is not a license to moan, groan, complain and constantly feel sorry for yourself!

## What are the negative aspects of telling others?

Along with all of the good can come some of the bad. In evaluating the two, we have found that the positive aspects of telling people outweigh the negative ones, but it is important to be aware that negatives do exist. Some people may respond very negatively to news that you have a serious illness. They may steer clear of you at work and avoid personal contact. This reaction can be very hurtful. Who knows why people react this way? It may be due to fear that you will become a burden to them or that they may have to pick up your slack if your disease causes you to reduce your level of activity. Whatever the reason, you must realize that nothing you do will make them feel differently. The best thing to do when this happens is to let go of the situation. If they really are your friends and were perhaps just stunned at your announcement, eventually they will come around. If they choose not to, it will be their loss.

## Assess Your Needs

When you were healthy and given a challenge, you called upon all of your available resources to successfully meet that challenge.

Being sick should make no difference in your approach. Think of yourself as an injured athlete in training for life's Olympics. As the star and captain of your wellness team it is your goal to put together a top-flight crew of experts selected for their ability to help you recuperate and win the gold!

Our recommended method for building your wellness team is best visualized as a circle in the middle of a blank piece of paper. Draw a circle and write your name in the center. Next, draw spokes coming out of the center, and on each spoke write down a function or aspect of support that you believe is important to your wellness program.

## Your Wellness Team

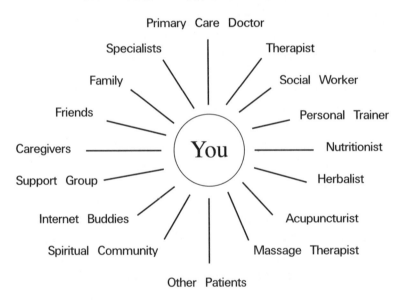

If you are married or have a family, you might write down that the love and support of your family is an important spoke in your wheel. Another important spoke might relate to the assistance that doctors can provide. Still other spokes may relate to the varied aspects of your professional and personal life. Allow for lots of spokes. You will be amazed at the number and breadth of things that come to mind. Once you have completed this step, then associate names of people who can provide you with needed assistance.

The first names that come to mind probably will be those to whom you are closest — your partner, immediate family, and possibly some dear friends. In addition to this "personal circle," you may choose to include the names of other relatives, friends and coworkers.

It should be fun and reassuring to think of everyone who is in a position to help you. However, it will take some forethought and organization to productively incorporate these people's efforts on your behalf. Without a plan, what begins with good intentions may end up as a mess of hurt feelings and frustration on all sides. To avoid this, first think about what you need done and how much help you will need, then ask people to assume responsibility for certain roles or to take on specific tasks.

For example, a spouse or adult child may be in the best position to handle communications for you during a medical crisis. He or she can screen your calls and provide information to others about your condition. Next, selected relatives may be able to help by doing research to locate the names of specialists and the latest information on treatment protocols relevant to your condition. Neighbors, friends, and coworkers can chip in by providing practical assistance such as running errands, taking care of your children and animals, cooking meals, and tying up loose ends in your personal and professional lives. And don't forget fellow patients who, because they can closely identify with your situation, may be able to provide you with a good laugh, much needed emotional support, and ideas and suggestions about how to get through your situation.

Although you are the captain of your team, you do not need to manage all of this coordination yourself. Assign the job to someone suited to the role and remember that team members can collaborate with one another. If, for example, you are looking for referrals to specialists, why not ask whoever is doing your medical research to talk with other team members for ideas?

If you are lucky enough to have more people willing to help than jobs needing to be done, let the volunteers know that you appreciate their offers of assistance and that someone will call them when you have a need. In many cases, people just want you to know that they care.

# Your Team of Doctors

## Your Primary Care Physician

Aside from your immediate family and friends, your next line of support is your primary care physician. She may have been involved in your care for some time and may have been the first to detect or identify your disease. Most likely, your primary care physician knows a lot about you and your medical history. She may be able to help you accomplish important tasks such as organizing and consolidating your medical records, facilitating referrals and approvals through your insurance carrier, helping you select the specialists who will be involved in your future care and coordinating their activities, as well as answering your medical questions. It is important to both respect and have confidence in your primary care physician. If you cannot trust and confide in your doctor, a change may be in order. However, depending on the immediacy of your need for treatment, you may be best served by staying with your current physician for the time being. Once your situation has stabilized, you can embark upon a search for a more suitable primary care physician.

## Specialists

The roster of specialists who join your wellness team is also very important. Depending upon your particular diagnosis, this roster may include surgeons, pathologists, radiologists, oncologists, cardiologists, gastroenterologists, neurologists, rheumatologists, and so on. The list may seem endless.

Your first introduction to a specialist usually comes at the recommendation of your primary care physician. Therefore, the better your primary care physician knows you, the better chance he has of suggesting a specialist who will be a good match for your specific needs and personal style.

It is not practical or necessary to feel as though you must have a close personal relationship with all of the specialists involved in your care. Although in some circumstances you may want to meet with the pathologist or radiologist who interpreted your tests, this is usually not necessary, nor is it a regular practice. What is most important in these instances is having access to the best minds available.

Whether it is necessary to feel emotionally connected to the surgeon or other specialist involved in your ongoing care varies from patient to patient. Many who are supported by positive relationships elsewhere do not feel it is imperative to mesh with a specialist's personal style. For some, it is enough to be treated by a doctor who is considered technically excellent. The fact that he may not come with an empathetic bedside manner is irrelevant. For others, rapport makes a critical difference. Only you can decide whether or not a specialist is a good match for you. Below are some tips to ensure that you and your specialists get off to a productive start.

## Things to Do When First Meeting with a Specialist

- Ask that your first visit be a "consultation." Tell the person making the appointment that you would like to "interview" or talk with the doctor about taking on your care. Some doctors will even provide this "introductory" service without charge.
- Try to establish this doctor's modus operandi. Ask him how he best likes to work with patients. Ask him how he views his role as compared to yours. His answers should tell you something about his personal style.
- Find the answers to practical matters such as how his office operates, how communications are handled within the office and to whom you should address your questions and needs on an ongoing basis.
- Try to get a sense of the availability of this doctor. Is he in or out of the office a lot? Does he regularly return phone calls from patients? If so, when (for example, at the beginning or end of the day)?
- Find out who in the office handles emergencies when the doctor is away.

# Other Practitioners

No matter how important your doctors are to your care, they can offer you only one facet of the assistance you need. There still remains a wealth of resources outside of these more traditional roles — resources that can make an important difference in how you feel. For you to truly get better in a holistic sense, you may need to expand your understanding of wellness. As part of this expanded awareness, be ready to broaden your scope. Open up your heart and your mind to accept the good things that a whole cast of others has to offer.

Other practitioners whose assistance you should consider include psychotherapists to help you deal with the emotional aspects of your disease, homeopathic experts, herbalists, acupuncturists, massage therapists, meditation specialists, physical therapists and trainers. These experts can help to relieve disease symptoms and improve your overall level of health with complementary therapies, and assist you in developing a stronger sense of body image and well-being. Your disease affects all of you. Therefore, the most productive approach involves treating your whole person, not just one isolated aspect of your being.

# Support Groups

For many patients support groups rank near the top of their list of most important resources. There is something about being able to share your questions, frustrations, fears and joy with others who are going through the same or similar experiences. Those who participate in support groups can offer a perspective and a wealth of collective knowledge that is almost impossible to find from any other single source. Try one out. They are well worth a visit, even if you don't think you are cut out for this type of therapy.

> *I sat in the surgical oncologist's room and couldn't believe what I was hearing. One week earlier, the doctor had performed a lumpectomy which confirmed breast cancer, and now he was going over the results of a lung biopsy — adeno-carcinoma in left mid-lobe with possible metastatic disease to*

*the periphery of the lung. Furthermore, he and my primary care physician were telling me that my bone scan indicated a possible tumor on the spine. How could this be? I'd never had any symptoms! Two months ago I was scuba diving and regularly performing single tank dive times over one hour — with lung cancer! I gritted my teeth and fought back the tears. It was at that point that my husband and I met the clinical social coordinator who moderated a weekly cancer support group. She invited us to come to a meeting. That support group played a primary role in saving my life — right up there with my hematological, radiological, and surgical oncologists.*

*I went through about two years of diagnosis along with surgery, chemotherapy, and radiation treatment. We could not possibly have foreseen or adequately prepared for the medical and non-medical problems we faced. However, over a short period of time, we came to realize that (collectively) the group members had experienced similar problems, and some of the information communicated during support group meetings helped us solve or even avoid problems. Communication is a key word, but that doesn't fully describe it — it's dynamic communication with sharing, caring, and understanding from your fellow cancer survivors. It provides real-time information which sometimes is concurrent with your diagnosis, treatment, and non-medical problems. This isn't available from books, tapes, news media, the Internet, or even your care providers.*

*I am now over one year in remission, and give my cancer support group a large share of the credit.*

Sally

Both of us have participated in support groups at different stages in our disease histories. We drop in and out of them as our needs warrant. Many patients get the most out of their support group experiences if they attend them while going through active treatment. Others don't feel the need to connect until after their treatments are over and they suddenly feel alone and adrift, having been released from the routine of supervised day-to-day care.

Today, many support groups emphasize a focus on and exploration of the self, incorporating approaches such as meditation, Eastern spiritual practices and T'ai Chi.

Support groups are no longer just for patients. More and more groups are now addressing the needs of spouses, children and caregivers during all phases of coping, grief and loss.

To find out about support groups, inquire at your doctor's office and check with friends. Call your local branch of a national disease organization and look for notices posted at medical centers and on the Internet or America Online. Support groups have their own personalities, so be prepared to visit a few different groups before settling on one that fits your needs and personality.

## Those Closest to You — Your Personal Support Circle

Giving and receiving care are very personal and emotional experiences for everyone involved, especially for the caregiver. Many sign on to play this part expecting that it will be a selfless and clear demonstration of their affection for a loved one. Most, however, are unprepared for how exhausting, stressful, and devoid of appreciation caregiving can be.

Caregivers have to cope with their own sense of grief about what is happening to a dear one, and also sometimes face a growing sense of resentment about how their actions are being perceived. Illness can turn even the sweetest people into difficult patients — and if loved ones were not so sweet to start out with, then caregivers can really find their hands full.

## To Caregivers

There are no hard and fast rules about how to be a good patient or caregiver. As patients ourselves, however, we can offer caregivers a few words of wisdom and advice:

- Regardless of what your patient says, he probably appreciates and depends on what you do.
- Understand that your patient will not be "up" all of the time. Allow him to occasionally explode. Do not take everything your patient says or does personally.

- Be clear with your patient. Tell her what you need from from her and what you will and will not do. Work to set guidelines of behavior and "time outs" — and don't feel bad when you say you've "had enough" or that you need to go. Tell your patient when she is being unreasonably difficult.
- Give your patient a role in his own care. Help him to get organized and feel as if he is taking charge of his situation. Do not insist on doing everything for him.
- Coordinate your efforts with others who are also assisting. Competition among caregivers does nothing to help the patient or the situation.
- Keep in mind that sometimes too much information is both overwhelming and confusing. Help your patient grasp information by providing it in bits and don't get impatient if you have to keep reminding her about something you have already said.
- Do not rush your patient into making treatment decisions. Generally, there is adequate time for reflection. It is very important that patients get comfortable with choices affecting their health and their quality of life.
- Allow your patient to make choices that fit his own personal style. Feel free to make known your ideas and recommendations, but do not be upset if your patient does not follow them.
- You may have to put your emotional needs on the back burner so you can help the patient with her immediate problems.
- Take good care of yourself. Your health and well-being are important, too.

# Chapter Eight

# Lifestyle Modifications

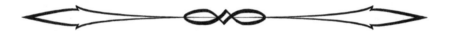

*I always considered myself to be an "up" person. For me, the glass was always half full, no matter what challenges life had to offer. However, when I finally realized that my disease was not going to go away, my spirits plummeted. At first, I wasn't even aware of the change in my outlook. Only my twin sister could see what was happening, and she urged me to get professional help. I didn't heed her advice for a long time. In fact, by the time I finally went to see a therapist, I was so down that I welcomed the prospect that my life would soon end. It was only with the help of an expert that I was able to summon the will to live.*

*Now, four years and three operations later, I am truly grateful for this assistance. I realize now that I could not have overcome my depression without professional help — and to have refused it would have meant death. Bolstered with a renewed sense of spirit, I used the Internet to search for a doctor who could help me live. Not only did I find one, but gradually I also rediscovered the joy in living. I have found satisfying meaning in my life even though my disease keeps recurring, and my lifestyle is much changed from my days as a business executive. Although it is not the life that I thought I would lead, it is a wonderful and, in many ways, much more meaningful existence.*

Alice

## Little Things Become Big

When you have a serious condition, even the small stuff feels like a big deal. Not only do you find it impossible not to sweat the little things, you also feel like you are on a constantly running emotional roller coaster. Even if you are able to present a stoic front on the outside, inside you may be in turmoil and sensitive to absolutely everything happening around you. Seemingly inconsequential occurrences can bring you down like never before. What used to be easily forgettable incidents now loom as life-stopping events.

Learning to cope with newfound emotions can be difficult, frustrating and extremely embarrassing. You may feel down-in-the-dumps now, even if you never have before. In this chapter, we address some important psychosocial issues that may affect you.

As much as you may want to discount its impact, your disease will have an everlasting effect on you. It is a life-changing event. Even if you go on to enjoy a full recovery, you will always carry this experience with you.

## This Experience Will Change Your Life

Be prepared! Your emotions will go up and down like a roller coaster ride. Even the most stoic people will go through some sort of emotional upheaval. Although each person's experience will be different, our advice is to go with the flow. Trying to stop the flood of emotions is fruitless and requires too much negative energy. Instead, allow your feelings to wash over rather than envelop you. Try to understand what is happening and why you feel as you do. You don't have to relish the process, but do your best to work through your emotions and then move on.

For many, denial is the first reaction. Sometimes it surfaces as outright rejection of the notion of even being ill. Others try to deny that their disease will impact their life and those around them. These are very normal reactions. So are anger, sadness and guilt. Sometimes, these feelings actually turn out to be positive responses, because in the short term they empower us with the energy needed to get through difficult aspects of our disease experience.

Some of us never get beyond these initial stages of emotion — especially when their diseases are limited to relatively short time spans with clearly identifiable cycles of diagnosis, treatment and recovery. For others, the odyssey is not so cut and dried. Do your best to work through your feelings. Try not to get stuck in any one emotion. Your goal should be to move through the negative ones as quickly as possible, so that you can get to ones that will be more conducive to your healing process.

## Attitude Is Everything!

The following anecdote says it all:

*Jerry was the kind of guy you love to hate. He was always in a good mood and always had something positive to say. When someone would ask him how he was doing, he would reply, "If I were any better, I would be twins!"*

*As a restaurant executive, he was a unique manager because he had several waiters who followed him around from restaurant to restaurant. The reason they followed was because of his attitude. Jerry was a natural motivator. If an employee was having a bad day, Jerry would be right there encouraging the employee to look on the positive side. Seeing him in action really made me curious, so one day I went up to Jerry and asked him, "I don't get it! You can't be a positive person all of the time. How do you do it?"*

*Jerry replied, "Each morning I wake up and say to myself, 'Jerry, you have two choices today. You can choose to be in a good mood or you can choose to be in a bad mood.' I choose to be in a good mood. Each time something bad happens, I can choose to be a victim or I can choose to learn from it. I choose to learn from it. Every time someone comes to me complaining, I can choose to accept their complaining, or I can point out the positive side of life."*

*"Yeah, right, but it's not that easy," I protested.*

*"Yes it is," Jerry said. "Life is all about choices. When you cut away all of the junk, every situation is a choice. You choose how to react to situations. You choose how people will affect your mood. You choose to be in a good mood or bad mood. The bottom line is that it's your choice how you live life."*

*I reflected on what Jerry said. Soon thereafter, I left the restaurant industry to start my own business. We lost touch, but often I thought about him whenever I made a choice about life instead of reacting to it. Several years later, I heard that Jerry did something you are never supposed to do in the restaurant business: he left the back door open one morning and was held up at gunpoint by three armed robbers. While he was trying to open the safe, his hand slipped. The robbers panicked and shot him. Luckily, Jerry was found relatively quickly and rushed to the local trauma center.*

*After eighteen hours of surgery and weeks of intensive care, Jerry was released from the hospital with fragments of bullets still in his body. I saw Jerry about six months after the accident. When I asked him how he was, he replied, "If I were any better, I'd be twins. Wanna see my scars?"*

*I declined to see his wounds but did ask him what had gone through his mind as the robbery took place. "The first thing that went through my mind was that I should have locked the back door," Jerry replied. "Then as I lay on the floor, I remembered that I had two choices: I could choose to live or I could choose to die. I chose to live."*

*"Weren't you scared? Did you lose consciousness?" I asked.*

*Jerry continued, "The paramedics were great. They kept telling me I was going to be okay. But, when they wheeled me into the emergency room and I saw the expressions on the faces of the doctors and nurses, I got really scared. In their eyes I read, 'He's a dead man.' I knew I needed to take action."*

*"What did you do?" I asked.*

*"Well, there was a big, burly nurse shouting questions at me," said Jerry. "She asked me if I was allergic to anything. 'Yes,' I replied. The doctors and nurses stopped working as they waited for my reply. I took a deep breath and yelled, 'Bullets!' Over their laughter, I told them I was choosing to live. 'Operate on me as if I am alive, not dead.' "*

*Jerry lived, thanks to the skill of his doctors and his own amazing attitude. I learned from him that every day we have the choice to live life fully. Attitude, after all, is everything.*

Francie

We are all given the opportunity to choose how we respond to our situations. Although we cannot change the fact that we are sick, we can choose to keep it from negatively affecting the rest of our lives.

## Thirteen Effective Ways to Modify Your Behavior

### 1. Forget guilt and blame.

Do not allow yourself to become overcome by guilt or obsessed with trying to assign blame for your situation.

Even if you made earlier lifestyle decisions that contributed to your present condition, you certainly did not intend to make yourself sick. Feeling guilty about your situation or blaming someone else for what is happening will not help you effect positive changes in your life. If others try to get you to behave this way, it is probably because something in their own lives is not quite right. Don't make their problems yours!

### 2. Be honest about how you feel.

Be honest with yourself and others about your feelings. Refusing to acknowledge your emotions will not make them go away. If you feel angry or depressed (and you will), be honest enough to say, "I'm angry, or I'm depressed, about what is happening to me right now." Then do your best to work through these feelings. Sometimes, admitting that you have these emotions goes a long way toward letting them go.

### 3. Accept that your situation has changed.

You will not be able to create a more positive emotional outcome until you accept that your life is changing. Acceptance doesn't mean you have to embrace the role of "sick person." Acceptance means fully acknowledging where you stand, both physically and emotionally, so that you can move on and develop a plan to battle your disease with the very best that both medicine and *you* have to offer.

Face reality, and then use your changing situation as an opportunity to try new things — or at least approach life with a new perspective. Don't miss a truly great opportunity. For all of the negative aspects of your disease, learning to embrace change can be one of the most positive things to come out of your situation. What a shame not to seize the opportunity!

### 4. Be prepared to make changes.

As you change, so does your relationship with everything and everyone around you. Do not be afraid of this. As you grow in your own awareness, so will your relationships with others. Unfortunately, sometimes old relationships turn out to be toxic elements in your new life. If being with someone makes you feel more ill than well, let them go. Maintaining ties with "toxic" friends makes it much harder to get well.

### 5. Seek professional help.

It is well documented that disease and its accompanying treatments can make you clinically depressed. Don't make yourself feel worse by thinking you should work through your emotions all by yourself. If you are consulting doctors to help heal your body, why not seek expert assistance to heal your spirit? Even if you are surrounded by supportive family and friends, the help of a professional can enable you to more easily move out of a difficult emotional place and get on with the process of healing.

## 6. Never underestimate the power of prayer.

Many patients find strength and peace through spirituality or prayer. Getting well is all about opening your heart as well as your body. Let the power of all healing influences help you.

## 7. Don't sweat the small stuff.

Don't let the little things in life trip you up and bring you down. If your morning didn't go well, if a relative is upset because you didn't come to dinner, or if you have to wait for an appointment with your doctor, don't allow these small things to irritate or upset you. Save your strength to weather the big storms. Don't waste energy on life's little squalls. Let go of the unimportant, and you will experience more joy in your days.

## 8. Have a sense of humor.

Laughing will make you feel better. If you don't believe us, there are studies that validate this claim. Maintaining a sense of humor, even in the worst of circumstances, can pull you through the really tough times.

## 9. Establish balance in your life.

Every day is a new day. One day you may feel good and the next may find you in the hospital. The truth is you may never again feel as physically good as you did before your illness, but that doesn't mean that you always have to feel bad.

Find a new level within yourself where you *do* feel good, and adjust your daily life to maintain that "feeling good" state. If your illness affects your digestion, for example, pay attention to basics like altering your diet or exercising regularly. If you have a heart problem, this may mean you have to restrict your activity so that your heart rate doesn't go above a certain level. Whatever your situation, find what you can do on a regular basis to keep feeling good.

Many people achieve balance by learning to relax through meditation or some other way such as deep breathing or visualization. Learning to let go for even a few minutes each day can create a greater feeling of peace and acceptance of your situation, which in itself can be very healing.

## 10. Bring joy into your life.

Smell the roses, go to the beach, eat your favorite dessert, cuddle your dog or cat. Do things that really satisfy you. Fill yourself with joy — joy so strong that the emotion helps you feel better. We are not espousing a New-Age-feel-good cure, but we have found that those who find ways to feel good in spite of their medical situations seem to be a lot more successful in overcoming the handicaps of their illnesses.

Your goal is to live a full and satisfying life, in spite of your disease and its possible physical limitations. Get comfortable with your life's new tempo. Don't let the fact that you must remain on the ground in the physical sense prevent you from soaring with the eagles in mind and spirit.

## 11. When you have something good to say, say it.

There's no time like the present. Don't keep your loving thoughts to yourself. Make every moment special and share your positive feelings with those around you. Don't wait until it is too late to tell your spouse, your parents, or your children how much you love them. If you are happy that your best friend came to visit, tell her. Let her know how much her friendship means to you. You will be amazed how much you get back when you open your heart up to those whom you cherish.

## 12. Don't be a complainer.

Acknowledge your limitations, but don't use them as an excuse to become a bore. Although most everyone will try to be sympathetic to your situation, no one likes to be around a negative person.

When someone asks how you are, don't unleash a litany of everything that ails you. Otherwise, even your closest friends will stay away. Most people ask because they want to appear empathetic. Do your best to respond in a straightforward yet brief manner, and try to convey a positive attitude. Saying something like, "I've had a difficult week, but tomorrow's another day, and I hope by then I'll feel better," is honest yet hopeful, and allows you both to move on to more engaging conversation.

## 13. Choose the ways you rebel.

Sometimes a little rebellion can be empowering if you feel a strong urge to strike back at your situation. Just make certain that you are not truly endangering your health by doing so. Canceling all your doctor appointments may not be a good idea. On the other hand, enjoying an occasional slice of pie may not completely undo your nutritional program.

# Chapter Nine

# Tests, Procedures and Your Medical Records

*After my oncology appointment, I happened to mention to one of the nurses that I was scheduled to have a catheter inserted in my chest. She asked me who was scheduled to do the procedure. When I told her, she said, "Oh no," and asked me to wait a few minutes while she went to talk with my doctor. When she returned, she explained that, although the doctor who was scheduled to perform the insertion was very good, she thought that another doctor would be better for me, because he was very successful at placing devices in ways that could be hidden by clothing, and the scars from his incisions were usually less visible. She thought I would be happier with the long-term results with the second physician. With permission from my oncologist, she changed my appointment and set me up with her recommended surgeon.*

*Now every time I put on an open-neck blouse or sweater, I am enormously grateful for her intervention. Unfortunately, she and my doctors failed to prepare me for the chest pain that*

*followed the surgery. I had to discover that for myself — but it
taught me an excellent lesson: Ask questions up front.*

Alice

## Tests and Procedures

The terms "test" and "procedure" are often used during your evaluation, treatment and follow-up. Sometimes they are used interchange-
ably. Don't get hung up on the distinctions. Either way, something is
being *done* to you.

You will undergo what may seem like an endless array of medical
tests and procedures, not only in the diagnostic phase of your illness,
but throughout the course of your treatment and follow-up.

Tests and procedures are necessary to help your doctor determine
the origins of your medical problem, confirm a preliminary diagnosis,
or determine the effects and side effects of treatment. They may also be
used to evaluate the changes in your illness over a period of time.

While your doctor may downplay the impact of a given test or
procedure, it is important to have a clear understanding of what is involved,
and the expected risks and benefits, before you agree to anything.
Remember that you will be the one affected by whatever is done.

Whenever possible, talk with others who have already undergone
the proposed test or procedure, or ask a nurse or lab technician for
information before you submit to anything. Your doctor or the test
facility may have books and pamphlets about the test or procedure.
Know what to expect about the process, the anticipated results, and any
consequences or side effects you may face.

## Questions to Ask

Here are sixteen questions you should consider asking before
undergoing any test or procedure:
1.   Why this test or procedure?
2.   Is it really necessary?
3.   What will happen if it is *not* done?
4.   What risks are involved?

5.   What sort of preparation is needed?
6.   What will happen during the test or procedure?
7.   How will I feel during and after the test or procedure?
8.   Is there an alternative test or procedure or any variation in the way it is administered that I should know about?
9.   What is the expected outcome?
10.  What will the results show?
11.  How will the results affect me, my diagnosis, or my treatment?
12.  How and when will I find out about the results?
13.  Who will explain the results to me?
14.  Who will answer any questions I might have later?
15.  Where will the record of my test or procedure be stored?
16.  How and when can I obtain a copy of this record?

## Considerations in the Selection of Tests

Doctors differ on the kinds of tests and procedures they use. One may administer a CT scan while another orders an ultrasound to learn about the same condition. In some instances the same test or procedure can be used for a variety of purposes. Blood tests, for example, can be used to study or determine a wide range of illnesses. Some tests provide only partial answers, whereas others paint a more complete picture.

Costs and insurance considerations, as well as the health of the patient, may help to determine which test is administered. Some tests are less invasive or risky than others, and your doctor may elect the method that has the least impact on you. Ask your doctor to explain his testing strategy. The important thing is to know as much as possible about your options, so you can help your doctor match the appropriate test to your situation and needs.

Often your doctor will start out with a simple, selective test and then order more if the results indicate the need.

Doctors don't always make decisions that consider your individual desires, needs or comfort. Your doctor may be accustomed to having a test done in a particular way or at a specific location, even though several options may exist. The medical center or your insurance company may prefer certain tests or methods, or your doctor may prefer a specific lab or specialist to perform the procedure. Even though your doctor may have good reasons for his choices, they may not be right for you. Here are some examples:

Your doctor orders a CT scan of your abdomen, which requires that you drink copious amounts of an unpleasant liquid called a diagnostic solution. For some, the result is nausea, vomiting or diarrhea. But if you took the time to learn about CT scans, you would find that not all CT scanners and diagnostic solutions are identical. The newer CT machines take less time to complete a procedure and there are several available brands of diagnostic solutions — each with a different flavor and consistency. These options can make a big difference in how you feel during and after your test. In some cases, you won't have a choice about where the test is administered or which brand of diagnostic solution is used, but you never know unless you ask.

MRI scans are another good example. Patients with claustrophobia dread the MRI experience because they think they'll have to lie perfectly still for long periods of time in an enclosed capsule. But many facilities now offer "open MRIs" that avoid the problem, or will administer you a mild sedative on request to reduce your uneasiness.

A third example involves the insertion of catheters (thin tubes) into your arm, chest, or other parts of your body. This can cause problems for some people. Catheters are a necessary part of some treatments for cancer, infections, and diabetes. Many doctors will tell you that the insertion procedure is "a piece of cake." Maybe from their point of view. What you may not be told is that, depending on the doctor's skill and where he places your catheter, the insertion can leave you with an unsightly plastic tube hanging from a very visible and uncomfortable place on your body, as well as an unwanted permanent scar after the tube is removed. After the anesthetic wears off, you may experience a great deal of pain and discomfort for as long as three to five days! Some surgeons are better at some procedures than others.

The lesson to be learned is: Remember to ask about all your options.

# When You Go for Your Test or Procedure

"Hurry up and wait" describes the experience of many who undergo lots of tests and procedures. Always go prepared with plenty of your favorite reading material, and remember to dress comfortably for your visit. Even if you're not the "sweatpants and sneakers" type, keep in mind that you will spend inordinate amounts of time waiting in uncomfortable chairs. Procedure rooms are often freezing cold, and you will usually be asked to strip down completely and put on a thin cotton hospital gown. Find out if this indignity is really necessary. If not, keep on as many clothes as possible. Being cold causes your veins to run for cover, making them impossible to locate when needed, and it adds to your already increasing sense of uneasiness.

Be stubborn! Why must you remove your pants and underwear when they are taking X-rays of your breasts? Appeal to the technician's common sense. However, if you must "bare all," at least bring a cap to keep your head warm or wrap your sweatshirt around you to comfort you while you wait. Being comfortable will help you relax. Once you get into the examination room, the technician will sometimes offer you a warm blanket. Be greedy! If you are cold, ask for at least two, because the heat from the first may wear off after a few minutes, leaving you to shiver through the rest of the procedure.

# Ask for a Copy of Your Report

If a report is issued following your test or procedure, be sure to obtain a copy for your own information and files. The most effective way to be certain that a report is sent to you is to have the doctor who requests the procedure stipulate on the form everyone who should receive a copy, including you. Another way is to have someone in your doctor's office fax or send the report to you after they receive their copy. Some doctors like to have you meet with them to receive and discuss your report findings. Others will send you a copy prior to or in lieu of an office visit. A doctor's decision is based on his personal style and his understanding of your preferences and the importance of a particular test or procedure to your overall diagnosis or treatment. We both prefer to obtain copies of our reports prior to meeting with our doctors, so that we can do our homework ahead of time. We circle all the words or phrases we don't recognize, and then we do our best to gain an understanding of them before we see our doctors. By preparing in advance for our visits, we are able to use the doctor's time more effectively and to our advantage.

Be careful not to let information in the report overly frighten you. Many people get scared by what they read because it sounds so clinical and depressing or because they have no idea what it all means. Preventing unnecessary fear or worry is one reason why doctors like to review report findings with their patients, especially newly diagnosed individuals. The specialist directing the test or procedure is responsible to call out everything she finds. For long-term patients especially, reports can be full of scary-sounding but otherwise benign information. Alice, for example, has undergone surgeries and chemotherapies that left long-term scars on her organs and damaged her liver. These scars are noted in detail on every new CT scan, even though they are not indicative of a disease recurrence or progression. Here is a case where a medical-expert friend might help allay your concerns.

## When You and Your Doctor Disagree

You and your doctor may occasionally disagree about your need to undergo a test or procedure. When this happens, listen carefully to what she has to say, and then make your own determination. If your body is sending you strong messages that something is wrong, yet your doctor is unable to confirm your feelings by simple tests, you may want to press for something more extensive. In some cases you may have to pay the full cost of the procedure because your insurance will not approve it. Paying out of your own pocket will cause you to think long and hard about the expected benefits. If you still believe that the test is the right way to go, get a second opinion, then shoulder the expense yourself or prepare to challenge your insurance company.

Your doctor may also want to perform a test or procedure that you don't want. This issue comes up in cases where you have decided not to undergo a specific treatment, such as chemotherapy or radiation for cancer, and your doctor wants to ascertain if your disease has continued to spread. What will be the benefit if you agree to go ahead with the recommended test or procedure? Will it change your mind regarding treatment? Will it make a difference regarding future decisions about your overall care? If the benefits are not clearly apparent after you obtain appropriate advice and consultation, we say, "Don't do it."

## Your Medical Records

*I enrolled in Mary and Alice's class on "How To Be Your Own Patient Advocate." It was at a time in my life when I could no longer bury my head in the sand about my personal health. These two women had many good ideas, and I was especially struck by the suggestion that my medical records could and should be made available to me by my doctor.*

*I thought to myself, "This is something I can do!" I resolved to call my doctor and ask him for copies of my records. Then I thought, "It can't be that simple. What would my doctor think? Would he think I was unhappy with his care? Would he think I was going to sue him? Would he still be willing to be my doctor if I asked him for the information?"*

*The more I thought about it, the more hesitant I became. Although I had once thought getting the records was a good idea, my fears overcame my enthusiasm and I kept putting it off.*

*Some months later I saw Mary, and she asked if I had gotten my records. Not wanting to admit what was really going on, I replied, "Not yet."*

*"Do you want me to help you make the call?" she asked.*

*"Give me two weeks," I said. "If I haven't done it by then, I'll take you up on your offer."*

*A few days later I gathered up my courage, called my doctor's very busy office and asked to speak to his assistant. "I'd like a copy of my medical records and I'd..."*

*"Just a second," she interrupted cheerfully, "and I'll connect you with Fred."*

*When Fred came on the line, I made the same request of him. "No problem," he said. "I will call you when it's ready."*
*And he did call the very next day.*
*Wow! What a sense of empowerment I felt. Next time I won't take so long to act.*

Doris

The term "medical records" refers to all of the information that is stored about you as a patient. This information includes reports (such as pathology, surgery and doctors' reports, as well as correspondence), slides, X-rays, scans and videotapes. Records are stored in a variety of places (hospitals, treatment centers, doctors' offices, etc.), which is why you need to take responsibility for keeping track of them. Records are not kept forever. Although the actual record does not belong to you, generally you have access rights.

Researching and maintaining all of this information can be time consuming and frustrating, especially if you have visited several different doctors and medical centers. The best time to begin record keeping is while you are healthy or as soon as you become aware that you have a medical problem. To keep track of your medical records, you will need to know where each record is kept and its medical record number. You will also need to know how to obtain copies of your records. Procurement procedures vary from state to state and from one medical center to the next. Most, however, will require at least the following information. Make several copies to keep on hand.

---

## Test/Procedure Record

Type of procedure/test: _____

Date and location where performed:_____

_____

Contact office and/or name: _____

Phone #: _____ Fax #: _____

Medical record #: _____

Doctor who ordered the test/procedure: _____

---

Whenever possible, secure copies of all written records for your own files. Ask a staff person in your doctor's or hospital's medical records office how to gain access. In some cases you may be asked to sign a medical records release form and pay a copying fee.

Sometimes it is more expedient to have a medical record released to your doctor, who can pass it along to you, such as when your record is in the form of a slide or X-ray. However, many medical centers and hospitals are now used to patients asking for direct access to slides and X-rays.

To learn more about the laws in your state pertaining to medical records, write for the following seventy-four-page booklet:

*Medical Records — Getting Yours: A Consumer's Guide to Obtaining and Understanding Medical Records*
by Diann Johnson and Sidney Wolfe, M.D.
published by the Public Citizen's Health Resource Group
1600 20th Street, NW
Washington, DC 20009
(202) 588-1000
Send payment of $12.50 or call for credit card purchases.

# Chapter Ten

# How to Make the Most of Treatment Programs and Clinical Trials

*I have been in a pain trial now for more than a year. Initially I used the trial treatment as a total replacement for my previous pain medication, but it was inadequate. I had to get up every four hours to take a drug, and neither I nor my husband was getting enough sleep. After the trial was over, I switched to a new drug to treat breakthrough pain. Now I am back to using morphine on a regular basis and I only use the new medication when necessary. I will stay on this new treatment plan until the trial drug is licensed by the FDA. I keep a diary of all my health problems and of the efficacy of the new drug and send this information to the researchers.*

Pam

## Help Your Treatment Program Work for You

Treatment programs take on many different forms depending on your particular illness, as well as other factors such as your physical condition. Some remedies can be administered in the comfort of your own home, while others require time in a clinic or hospital. Although where you receive your treatment can make a big difference in how you feel about the therapy, don't let the environment negatively cloud your attitude. Here are eight things you can do to focus positive energy on making your treatment plan work for you:

## 1. Talk with others who have undergone similar therapies.

Other patients are your best "real life" resource for information about what the experience will be like. Not only can you get detailed information about the procedure, you can also get a "feeling" about what to expect and what to look out for.

## 2. Thoroughly familiarize yourself with your treatment surroundings before beginning your therapy.

If possible tour your treatment facility ahead of time and introduce yourself to the staff who will be assisting you. Get to know them on a personal basis before being admitted as a patient.

## 3. Understand what your treatment is supposed to accomplish, how long it should take for results, and how your progress will be measured.

Find out everything you can do to maximize the potential of your treatment, and how to deal with any side effects. Many patients use this treatment phase as an opportunity to explore complementary therapies to enhance their treatment and their overall sense of well-being. These include such practices and remedies as nutritional healing, herbs, acupuncture, massage, meditation, yoga and much more.

## 4. Prepare yourself both mentally and physically before your treatments.

Eat well, get plenty of rest, and ask your doctor for recommendations about what you can do to get yourself in tip-top shape for the procedure. Engage in your favorite activities before and after your treatments. In the days prior to your treatment, spend some quiet time thinking positively about what will happen. Visualize getting well. Write out meaningful affirmations and recite them before, during, and after each procedure.

## 5. Approach your initial treatment as a learning opportunity.

This is a chance for you to thoroughly understand the treatment experience you will be having. Take notes during (if possible) or soon after your first therapy session, to record anything you didn't like that you might be able to change. Do whatever is necessary to adapt your treatment environment to make it comfortable for you. If you must go into the hospital, bring a favorite shawl or blanket to cuddle up in and surround yourself with pictures of your loved ones. Bring along favorite music tapes or CDs to listen to while your treatment is being administered. If you don't want to be alone while receiving treatment, arrange to bring a buddy. If you love to play card games, bring a deck of cards along with your friend. If you must remain overnight and are afraid of being alone, ask whether someone can spend the night. For medical reasons, the answer may be no, but you'll never know unless you ask.

## 6. During and after your treatment, be alert to symptoms that don't seem right and notify your doctor as soon as you become aware of them.

Don't be surprised if your doctor is not completely interested in how you tolerate your treatment, unless it directly affects your medical condition. Nurses, friends and other professionals may be better able to help you work through side effects that are non-life-threatening or more emotional in nature.

## 7. Keep a journal or take notes about your treatment experiences.

Write down which devices, drugs and dosages are used, what you are thinking, and how you feel at every step along the way.

## 8. If your treatment is out of town, make certain your hometown doctors are up to date on how to evaluate and treat possible side effects.

Ask your treatment doctor to put information about your protocol in writing for you to carry with you when you return home. Not being prepared for potential emergencies can cost you your life.

*Like many cancer patients, I underwent specialized medical treatment at an institution away from home. Fortunately, the experienced team at Denver's University Hospital has many patients who return to local doctors for follow-up. With this in mind, before patients "leave the nest" the team thoroughly brainwashes them about what possible side effects and symptoms of complications to watch for, as well as what tests can confirm diagnosis and what treatments are available. I don't know if all doctors and clinics are this thorough, so it's a good general rule for any patient to ask such detailed questions before being released.*

*In my case, I went for a routine pulmonary function test when I returned home. The results of this and an exercise test showed every indication of toxic lung disease as it was explained to us in Denver. It is a common but serious side effect.*

*My local doctor, who had only treated the disease in its severe stages, felt there was nothing to be concerned about since I wasn't breathless. For a week my calls to him went unreturned; we communicated only via his nurse. I finally called the team in Denver, who collected the test results from my local hospital. They called back with urgent orders to pick up the required medication immediately and begin the ten-week detoxification. If not caught in time, this illness cannot be treated successfully and becomes a permanent condition.*

*One's local physician, regardless of how well-meaning, is not generally very experienced with the side-effect diseases common in specialized medical treatments. So, keep yourself informed and take control when necessary. Being aware and overly cautious enabled me to save myself from a possible miserable end.*

Sarah

# Clinical Trials

As part of any search for possible treatment options, it is important to know about scientific research that might pertain to your disease. Clinical trials offer insight into potential treatment breakthroughs, and participating in one is a tangible way to take advantage of cutting-edge scientific developments. Although not for everyone, clinical trials offer the most current medical thinking in therapy and patient care. They can be an especially welcome resource for those who have exhausted traditionally accepted methods of treatment. They are also sometimes used as the first line of treatment. Just because it involves new thinking, however, does not mean that a clinical trial is the best course for you to follow.

There are several ways to find out about available clinical trials. You can ask your doctors, of course, and other experts whose advice you have sought for second opinions. You can also find research information on the Internet. Web sites geared to specific diseases often contain links to pertinent trial information. Up-to-date listings can also be found through *MEDLINE* at http://medlineplus.nlm.nih.gov/medlineplus or through *Center-Watch* at http://www.centerwatch.com/. Internet mail lists, newsgroups and support groups also carry information about clinical trials.

Trials are often divided into three separate phases.

The purpose of Phase One is to determine the proper dose and to learn the toxic side effects of the treatment or drug under study. No evidence of efficacy in Phase One trials is required in order to proceed to Phase Two. Although clinically good results rarely occur in this phase, you may want to consider participating if you have no other alternatives.

Phase Two trials are intended to determine the treatment's range of efficacy. In the case of cancer, this means finding which cancers the treatment might be effective against. Phase One and Phase Two trials have no control groups. They are intended for situations where the standard treatments have failed or, occasionally, for individuals who have rejected the standard treatment.

In Phase Three trials the new remedy is tested against an established protocol. Control group(s) receive the standard treatment and everyone else receives the experimental one. As a result of Phase Three trials, the new treatment may replace an old one and become the new standard, or it may become a second-line option to be used when the regular treatment fails. Based on today's code of medical ethics, all patients in Phase Three trials receive some type of treatment. The only exception is when the standard treatment for a certain condition is "no treatment."

If it becomes obvious in any phase of a trial that the patients are not safe or that the treatment is not working, the trial will be stopped and the patients can be switched to something else. If all available means of treatment have been exhausted, patients can receive palliative care to at least be kept comfortable. The converse is also true. If at some point it becomes obvious that trial patients are faring far better than the control group, the trial will be halted and all patients switched to the new therapy.

When you discover a clinical trial that might interest you, call the research group for further information. All trials stipulate certain conditions for participant inclusion. Establish as early as possible whether you are qualified to be considered as an applicant. If you are, then carefully consider all the information you receive before deciding to participate. Here are four issues to think about before participating in a clinical trial.

## Clinical Trials: Issues to Consider

### The therapy might not work.

Any treatment might be ineffective, but with clinical trials, the point cannot be emphasized too strongly. By their very definition, clinical trials are unproven methods of treatment. The scientists have reason to believe that a certain therapy may prove beneficial or they wouldn't spend money testing their theory, but there is a big difference between theory and practice. Hoping that a new treatment will be successful is a good thing, but too much hope may be unrealistic and leave you feeling emotionally devastated if things don't work out according to your expectations.

**You can take the time you need to consider all aspects of a clinical trial.**

Don't let anyone rush you into signing up. Take some time to determine whether you really want to participate. Your doctor might be enthusiastic about your participation because your enrollment will benefit him, not necessarily because it is the best course for you.

**Participation in clinical trials is not always free.**

Some experimental therapies have costs associated that may not be covered by your insurance. Be sure to ask questions about the financial aspects of the trial.

**You are likely to receive lots of focused medical attention, especially if you are getting positive results.**

Even if you are not among those receiving the actual treatment under study, you stand an excellent chance of getting that treatment later if the overall test results prove positive. If you receive the test treatment and do not respond positively, the bad news is you may have to deal with unknown side effects, which might put you in a state of crisis. You also may feel the cold shoulder if your results are not what the researchers had hoped. They may not actually shun you, but as part of your own disappointment with the results, you may feel put off.

Participating in a clinical trial as a form of treatment is the right thing to do for many patients. Whether it is the best road for you can only be determined through careful research and consideration.

# Chapter Eleven

# Medications

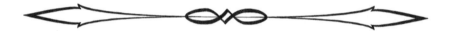

*It didn't even occur to me to pop the top off the bottle at the pharmacy before paying for the pills. After all, this was a refill of a prescription I had been getting there for a long time.*

*That night, however, I knew something was wrong when I removed the lid. These were not the same pills I was used to taking. Not only were they much larger than my regular ones, but they were of a different color.*

*Thank goodness for that, and for the fact that I still had a few pills left from my earlier prescription! The next day when I showed both sets of pills to the pharmacist, he looked up my latest prescription so we could read it together. Sure enough, the new prescription was slightly different from my old ones. My doctor and I had agreed that I would increase my overall daily dosage by taking the same pills more times per day. The pharmacist had misread the order and issued me pills that were each four times the strength of my old ones. If I had just started to take the new pills without paying attention, I could have suffered a serious overdose.*

Alice

Anything that you put into your body not only can have a direct effect, but also interacts with other things you consume.

As a patient, you must take responsibility for your own body. Be careful what you ingest, especially when it comes to medications. While you always hope to benefit from taking a medication, you also might suffer the consequences. Be aware of the effects, side effects, and possible interactions of every pharmaceutical prescription, herb or homeopathic remedy you take.

## Before You Begin Taking Any Medication

Learn all you can about every medication before you take it. Ask your pharmacist to talk with you about any new prescriptions. Ask for a copy of the drug company literature, which outlines everything you should know about the medicine. Before you take anything, read all the fine print. Be as critical of alternative medications as you are of mainstream drugs. Just because it is natural does not mean it is good for you.

### Questions to Ask Before Taking Medications

- What is the desired effect?
- How does it work?
- How long should it take to produce the full effect?
- What are the possible side effects and cautions?
- Does it interact with any other food or medication I'm taking? (This includes herbs and other non-prescription aids.)
- Does this new drug increase or decrease the effects of other medications?
- When should I take it and how? With or without food or drink?
- What effect will this drug have on other aspects of my life? For example, should I decrease my level of exercise or stay out of the sun when taking a certain medication?

You can obtain this information through your pharmacist, your doctor's office, books such as *The Physician's Desk Reference* (PDR) or drug manuals, or over the Internet. Two particularly good books are *The People's Pharmacy* and *Deadly Drug Interactions — The People's Pharmacy Guide,* both by Joe Graedon and Teresa Graedon, Ph.D.

Software programs are now available to help you organize and keep track of your medications. Parsons Technology offers one called "Medical Drug Reference 4.2". It can be ordered by telephone at (800) 548-1806 or over the Internet at http://www.parsonstech.com/home/medical.html.

## Keep Your Doctors Informed about Your Medications

Make sure all of your doctors know everything you are taking, and tell them about any previous drug reactions you have experienced. This information should be clearly highlighted on your medical resume form (see chapter 3), which you will have already given to your doctor. If you are unsure about your medications, carry all of them with you to your doctor's appointment. Don't transfer anything to a pill carrier, and don't simply bring samples of individual pills. Your doctor will need to see your medications in their original containers.

## Make a Friend of Your Pharmacist

Develop a working relationship with the pharmacists who fill your prescriptions. They often know more than your doctor about drugs and their interactions. After all, it's their specialty. It's a good idea to have all of your prescriptions filled at one pharmacy, so they can maintain an ongoing record of all of your medications. The big chains can to do this through networked computers.

You may want to consider ordering your medications through a mail order or online prescription service. These methods are especially convenient if you require consistent and ongoing delivery of specific drugs. Sometimes these services can even reduce your costs. Although you aren't able to meet with a pharmacist face to face in these circumstances, you can still communicate with one over the phone or by e-mail. Follow the same guidelines to make sure the provider is aware of everything you are taking, and always ask about possible interactions and side effects associated with any new prescription.

# Know Your Medications and When to Take Them

Become familiar with what your medications look like and what the dosages should be. Mistakes will still happen, no matter how many systems your pharmacy puts into place to prevent them. Get to know the size, color and shape of your medications. Pharmaceutical companies alter these aspects according to dosage to help the pharmacist, and you, be able to identify what you are getting. Read the label and pop the cap of any new prescription before leaving the pharmacy. If anything looks different about your medication from one prescription to the next, *do not take it* before checking with your pharmacist.

Many pills and capsules look alike, especially herbs and homeopathic medications. Don't pick up a loose pill from your countertop and pop it into your mouth unless you are absolutely certain what it is. This same caution applies to medications that are given to you in the hospital or doctor's office. Make certain that the type and dosage are right for you before agreeing to take anything. If you require reading glasses, be sure to use them to read any labels. When taking pills during the night, turn on a light and confirm that it is the correct medication before swallowing it.

Establish a schedule for taking your medications and stick to it. Experiment with timing to find a routine that works well for you. For example, you may have a pill to take at night, but discover that taking it right before lying down gives you indigestion. If this is the case, you may be better off taking it an hour before bedtime.

Many people find it hard to remember to take pills during a certain portion of the day, like noontime, when they often are busy and in the company of others. Establishing a habit will help you be consistent. Many products are available to help you, including automatic timing devices, dosage containers, and boxes with compartments divided to indicate different times and days.

*I participated in a support group with a lady who was taking large doses of antioxidants while she was receiving radiation therapy. She was having no side effects. When she told her doctor, he was very impressed and indicated he would mention it to his other patients. I was aghast. I could not believe that a radiation oncologist could be unaware that radiation therapy works by producing free radicals, which damage DNA and kill cells. If a patient takes a substance with the stated purpose of reducing free radicals, it may reduce damage to cells. In this particular case, however, damage to cells is the desired effect of the radiation treatment.*

*It is also true that some foods and herbs contain chemicals with hormonal effects, which might be harmful to someone whose cancer is affected by hormones. This is why it is so important to learn as much as possible about the nutritional and alternative products we consume.*

Pam

## While You Are on Medications

Pay attention to how your medications work. Make a note of any unexpected effects, and let your doctor know if they continue or are severe. Some people initially experience reactions to drugs, which gradually wear off as they get used to the medication. Make your doctor aware of any unexpected results. You can also call the drug company directly on their customer service lines to report any negative reactions. These telephone numbers are printed on the product literature, which you should always ask for with your prescription. If your medication does not have the desired effect after a reasonable time, talk with your doctor about alternatives.

Do not stop taking any medications without letting your doctor know. This includes herbal remedies, over-the-counter medicines, and prescription drugs. If your physician prescribed a medication knowing what else you were taking, then you should let him know whenever you change the mix.

In some cases, even your diet can have a serious effect on the drugs you consume. For example, the benefits of the anticoagulant drug Coumadin are diminished when you eat a lot of food high in vitamin K, such as broccoli and spinach. Consequently, patients taking Coumadin should have their blood checked regularly and continually adjust their medication and diet to continue deriving the greatest possible benefit from the drug.

## When You Travel

Make sure to plan ahead for your medical needs when you travel. In addition to a copy of your medical resume (see chapter 3), take extra pills along. Also, ask your doctor to write a prescription for small amounts of your medications, in case you lose your pills or stay away longer than expected. Carry pills and prescriptions as part of your hand luggage on the plane. Don't risk being separated from needed medications in case your baggage doesn't arrive on time.

Take responsibility for your well-being by becoming aware of what you put into your body. Work with your doctors and pharmacists to coordinate and manage your medications to your best advantage.

# Chapter Twelve

# Hospital Stays

*It was 10:30 in the morning and I felt awful. My tempera-*
*ture had risen steadily to an alarming 105 degrees. My doctor,*
*when he had heard how high my fever was, had ordered me to*
*get to the hospital as fast as possible. That alone was enough to*
*make me nervous, but now I had been in the hospital for over*
*an hour and was still waiting for treatment.*

*My wife was with me, trying her best to look brave. The*
*nurse in charge had been very helpful in getting me gowned and*
*assisting me with all the paperwork, but she didn't seem to*
*know much about my treatment.*

*"Nurse, do you know when I'll get my antibiotics?" I finally*
*asked.*

*"I'll see," she said. Twenty minutes later she returned.*
*"The pharmacy still has to make up the prescription."*

*"How long will that take?" I asked.*

*"About half an hour," she replied.*

*After the half hour passed, my wife said, "Call her back;*
*this is silly." This time the nurse informed me that an IV nurse*

*would have to put a tube in my arm and that the lab needed to draw blood before the antibiotics could be administered.*

*"When will the IV nurse be here?" I asked.*

*"I'll check," said the nurse in charge.*

*"I'll call the lab," said my wife.*

*I was trying my best not to be difficult, but I had now been waiting almost two hours for treatment. This time only twenty minutes went by before I pressed the call button again. "The IV nurse?" I asked.*

*"I called," responded the nurse in charge.*

*Finally, a full two-and-a-half hours after my admittance to the hospital, the IV nurse arrived, but the lab technician who was supposed to draw blood was nowhere to be found.*

*"I'm calling the doctor," my wife said. When she did, she found his office closed for lunch.*

*Eventually the lab technician did arrive and announced that she needed to draw blood from three separate sites. "Why three?" I asked.*

*"I don't know, but that's what's stated on the order," she said.*

*More than an hour after the lab technician finished stabbing me in the arm as well as the backs of both hands, the nurse returned triumphantly, carrying my first IV bag of antibiotics. She got it going just as my doctor walked into the room. He made a face when I told him that treatment had just begun.*

*"I didn't think it would take so long," he said. "Perhaps I should have written 'stat' on my admitting instructions."*

*I asked him why I had needed blood drawn from three separate locations. "Beats me," he said.*

*Just as I was beginning to relax, the nurse walked into the room and said, "They made up the wrong dose. The pharmacists only gave you half of what the doctor called for. They said they would send up a second bag soon."*

*Yikes!*

*Boy, did I learn a few lessons the hard way that day. Now I understand the importance of asking questions whenever I am in a situation concerning my health. I should have found out from my doctor what to expect* before *I went to the hospital. That way, when the delays and confusion began I could have called his office sooner, armed with the knowledge that things were not going as planned.*

*Once you are in the hospital, it is almost impossible to get the total picture. Everyone's duty is so specialized, and no one seems to have a grasp of the full view. That day I learned that you, the patient, must be in charge. In addition, I learned to ask the staff not just what comes next, but what comes after that. If they don't know, ask if there is someone else who does. Don't just lie there, ignorant and unhappy. Take responsibility for your own condition.*

Bill

Hospital stays, including visits to the emergency room, are common occurrences for many people with serious diseases. Although your experience probably differs from the one outlined above, there are several common things you can find out and be prepared for, especially in the case of emergencies.

Both of us have spent more time in hospitals than we care to remember. So that you might benefit from our combined experiences, here are some suggestions to help you through the ordeal. Especially if you are lucky enough to be able to anticipate your hospital stay, these recommendations will go a long way toward making your experience a positive one. Entering the hospital strong in mind and body will play an important part in how you feel when you leave.

## Bring Someone with You to Act as Your Advocate

By the time you find yourself needing to go to a hospital, your health is likely to have deteriorated. Therefore, it is imperative that someone accompany you to the hospital to act as your advocate. The advocate's duty is to act on your behalf concerning every aspect of your care.

In Bill's story above, his wife's job as advocate was to be assertive when timely treatment was not forthcoming. An advocate can also help you, the patient, feel as comfortable as possible in often difficult circumstances, and help the hospital staff understand your medical history and the events leading to your admittance. Most importantly, he or she will act as another set of eyes and ears, double-checking that the treatments ordered by your doctor are actually the ones being administered.

## Familiarize Yourself with What Will Be Done

**Have a clear understanding of the purpose of your stay and the benefits it will bring.**

Before you check in to the hospital, clearly understand why you need to go, how long you should plan to stay, and what the expected benefits are. In many cases, your doctor will recommend a hospital stay and refer you to a specialist who will be responsible for your care in the hospital or perform any necessary procedures. Gain a general understanding of what to expect before talking with your surgeon or other specialist. Many doctors and medical centers have pamphlets and, in some cases, videotapes available for this purpose. Learn the basic terminology and clinical steps involved, as well as why your doctor thinks this procedure will benefit you. When you meet with your surgeon, ask questions about any remaining issues or concerns.

**Talk with others who have undergone the same procedure.**

Medical professionals talk about hospital stays only in terms of the clinical aspects. Another patient, however, can tell you what to really expect. Try to locate and talk with others who have already undergone the same or a similar procedure. Don't be shy; probe as deeply with your questions as they will allow.

Here are some valuable questions to ask:
- How did you deal with your pre-hospital anxiety?
- How much pain were you in?
- What was it like when you woke up after surgery?
- Did you get depressed?

- How did you feel afterwards?
- What did you do to aid in your recovery?
- What things should I watch for?

# Prepare Yourself

**Think positive!**

It's important to prepare yourself mentally. Think positively about your upcoming hospital experience as a necessary step toward getting well. All athletes undergo grueling training and then compete before they can claim victory. The same applies to you. Think of your hospital stay as a positive means to a healthy outcome. Like the athlete, you must face difficult challenges to successfully accomplish your goals.

**Prepare yourself physically.**

Talk to your doctor before embarking on a physical exercise program. Exercise may not be recommended for everyone, especially if you are suffering from a heart or respiratory condition.

If your doctor gives you the okay and you can anticipate your hospital stay, begin exercising as soon as possible. If you have never exercised before, start with some simple stretches and then open your front door and start walking. Begin on flat surfaces and gradually work up to hills and steeper terrain. If possible, carry some small (one- or two-pound) hand weights with you. Your goal is to increase your aerobic capacity. If you are already used to walking, try a slow jog. Other beneficial exercises include swimming, rowing, aerobics and step exercises — anything that gets your heart pumping and increases your breathing capacity. Be sure to incorporate simple warm up and cool down stretches into your routine.

**Review past hospital experiences.**

If you have ever been hospitalized before, remember anything that will help you and your doctors this time. Are you allergic to any kind of medication? Did you vomit in the recovery room? Was your room too hot or too cold? Were you ultra-sensitive to certain tastes or smells? Did the odor of perfume worn by the nursing staff or flowers in the room bother you, or make you feel better? What about the telephone? Did you like having people call you, or did you prefer not to have your phone ring?

Use these past experiences to help you create the best possible experience this time. If you have never before stayed in a hospital, talk with friends who have and use their insights, along with the questions above, to fashion a positive mindset and establish an in-hospital environment that will be right for you.

## What to pack.

Hospital stays these days tend to be shorter than in the past. You probably will not need to pack a lot, but bringing the few items that are most important to you will make a big difference in how you feel. Although the weight of the clothing you bring may be influenced by the weather, try to pack only machine washable garments. If they get soiled, it is an easy task for someone to get them laundered and ready again.

Ask the pre-admit nurse for advice on what to pack. Here is our short list of suggested items:

Bring an easy-to-get-into robe. A front zip or wraparound style is best. You will need a pair of slippers, scuffs or other comfortable walking shoes. Items to keep you warm are also recommended, no matter what the weather outside. Include a cardigan style sweater, or a shawl or poncho, to wear around your shoulders. The latter are especially handy if you have IVs because they are sleeveless. If you tend to feel cold easily, include a favorite lap blanket and a cap or warm headband.

Bring a simple toilet kit containing toothpaste, a tooth brush, comb or hair brush, shampoo, shaving items, hand lotion and any other "must-haves." If make-up is important to you, bring some lipstick and mascara to help you feel and look better. Leave jewelry and other valuables at home.

Bring music, books on tape, and some light reading material, too. Keep in mind that your ability to focus may be limited during your hospital stay. If you like to work on games and puzzles, bring simpler versions than you would normally tackle. Drugs and other medications can make you feel "fuzzy in the head." Your goal is to get enjoyment out of your resting activities. If what you bring is too complicated, you will only get frustrated, which may make you feel worse or put you in a bad mood.

Don't forget to bring your medical resume and Living Will or Durable Power of Attorney for Healthcare. Give them to the hospital when you are admitted.

## Ask to meet with your anesthesiologist before surgery.

The anesthesiologist is the person who monitors your vital signs and ensures that your body functions optimally during surgery. For peace of mind, it is a good idea to meet with him prior to going under anesthesia. Ask whether he will be with you during your entire procedure or overseeing other patients at the same time. If the latter is the case, ask who will be looking out for your best interests in his absence. Ask him to explain how he intends to sedate you and be sure to tell him about any allergic reactions to drugs that you have. If nausea has been a problem for you on previous occasions, let him know. He may be able to give you something to avoid a repeat experience.

## Look for ways to conquer your fear.

Hospitals are scary places. The hours just before any kind of procedure can be nerve-wracking, especially when unknown doctors or nurses walk into your room and proceed to poke, prod and prick you with little or no explanation. In these circumstances, we have found that deep breathing goes a long way to help ease our fear. Take the time to learn the techniques before you go into the hospital. Attend a class or ask a friend to teach you. Those who used Lamaze during childbirth may recall how to use controlled breathing to calm and refocus yourself in the delivery room. The comfort of a hand to hold is also helpful in containing your fear — as long as the person whose hand you are holding is not more nervous than you are!

Many people replace their fear with visualization and positive affirmations. Imagine a place where you feel totally safe, calm and strong, and let yourself go. It need not be a place you have actually visited. It doesn't even have to be real. The important aspect is feeling good about being there. The same holds true with affirmations. Write some down before going into the hospital and recite them daily. Use these positive statements to put yourself into a frame of mind that will help as you go into surgery. Tell yourself that you feel calm and strong and that you are going to come out of your procedure with the strength and will to ensure a full recovery. If you like, give a copy of your affirmations to the anesthesiologist or nurse anesthetist and ask them to read them out loud while they are administering your medications.

Music is a powerful and effective aid for getting you through really scary procedures. Bring a portable cassette or CD player with you and when you feel your nerves start to jitter, put the headphones on and turn the volume up high enough to shut out everything else around you. Choose music that really stirs your soul and sing along if you like. Let the wonderful, soaring emotions that you feel while listening to your favorite music envelop your entire mind and body. These powerful feelings can help you get through some tough hospital experiences. We know some patients who ask their doctors to play certain music during surgery so they can experience the positive impact under anesthesia.

## While Recuperating in the Hospital

**Check your attitude.**

Keep in mind that you and the hospital staff are all on the same team — yours! Sometimes, it may seem as though everyone else is failing to do the things necessary to help you; but keep in mind that when you are confined to bed, you feel traumatized and uncomfortable, and you may be on a powerful medication. These feelings of stress and illness manifest themselves in little ways, such as thinking no one responds quickly enough when you press the nurse call button. In most cases, your nurse will respond within the hospital's established time guidelines. Just for your own information, ask the floor nurse or supervisor what those are. If you really start to feel like the staff is plotting against you, test out your suspicion. The next time you press the call button, use your watch to measure how long it takes someone to respond.

If you receive treatment at a teaching hospital, you may be asked for permission for more than one person to examine you. Your cooperation in this provides important educational opportunities for doctors-in-training. You do have the right, however, to limit how often you get prodded and poked like a guinea pig.

### Limit your requests to the important ones.

Help yourself and the nursing staff by trying to anticipate your needs and then limit your calls for assistance to those that really require their participation. If you call every half hour for things like ice chips or help washing your face, you will significantly limit the staff's ability to help all of the patients under their care. Someone may not respond quickly to your request because they are taking care of a critical emergency for another patient. Think about how you would feel if an attendant did not respond to your critical need because he was responding to a non-essential request from another patient. Nevertheless, do not hesitate to speak with the nurse or a supervisor if you repeatedly experience delays in getting necessary assistance.

### Have confidence in your team of medical professionals.

The staff at your hospital is a team of professionals representing the full range of medical care. They have been selected because they are good at what they do. Try to learn the names of those who care for you and greet them as you would any friendly acquaintance.

You may not appreciate everyone's individual work style — and that is fine. You are still their first priority and they are working in your best interest. While you may not like everything they do, keep in mind they are trying to help you get well.

The technician who comes in to draw blood at 10:00 P.M. or the nurse who wakes you up at midnight to take your vital signs did not wait until then to intentionally disturb your sleep. They may be operating based on explicit instructions from your doctor, and they have responsibilities that extend beyond you. They are doing their best to take care of everyone, including you.

The nurse who one morning helped you take a bath may tell you the next morning to do it yourself. She is not being mean; she simply knows that you will get better faster by doing things for yourself.

The doctor who takes you off all liquids — even ice chips — is not trying to see how unbearable he can make your hospital stay. He may be trying to reduce the drainage from your stomach, which in turn may help speed your recovery.

Some days it may seem as though everyone is working against you. This is not the case. At times like these, step back, relax, and remember that by working with a team, you are going to get well.

### Help the hospital staff protect you.

Help the nursing and technical staff protect you from human error by being very careful about the medications you take and the procedures you submit to as an in-hospital patient. Make certain that someone compares your wristband identification with the identity instructions on all medications before they are administered. Have the nurse tell you exactly what the drug is, why it is being given, and what the expected benefits are to you. Many medications are predispensed at a central pharmacy, so be sure to double-check that what you are getting is correct in all respects and is really intended for you. Do not go along with any procedure if you have questions. Some care providers may call you fussy, but better fussy than dead from an adverse reaction!

### Get active.

The more quickly you start doing things for yourself, the better you will feel and the sooner you will be able to leave the hospital. Start by brushing your teeth and washing your face in the mornings. Don't lie in bed all day — sit up and, if you are mobile, move to the guest chair next to your bed. When you get the go-ahead from your doctor, put on your robe and slippers and start walking around the ward. Don't stop at once or twice a day — challenge yourself! If you walked to the nurse's station in the morning, go a little farther in the afternoon. If you made two laps around the halls one day, aim for three or four the next. Walk to the guest area on your floor and sit there awhile. This is a good way to meet other patients and caregivers. The more you move around, the better you will feel and the faster your body is going to start working again. Every step you take will help you get out of the hospital and back to your own home.

**Try to relax.**

During your hospital stay you will more than likely feel agitated, uncomfortable, and lacking in good quality sleep. Meditating, day dreaming, and allowing your mind to relax will help you fall asleep more easily and enable your body to get the rest it needs. Relaxing will also help you cope with those long stretches of time when you feel blue and a bit lost over being in the hospital. Listening to music, audio tapes and the radio, and watching television help a lot of patients. For some, praying and meditation can also be beneficial. Ask the nurse or staff social worker to request a counselor or member of the clergy to visit.

If massage or some other form of physical therapy would benefit you, ask your doctor to order it. If your insurance doesn't cover such treatment, you may have to make your own arrangements.

## Personal Caregivers

Personal caregivers are a necessary component of your wellness team. Most often these are family members or dear friends. Because today's hospital environments are much more intense and tend to be leaner in staff than in the past, you should do everything possible to have at least one personal caregiver with you as much as possible during your hospital stay. For many people, personal caregivers are their most important allies in getting well. They know you better than anyone else and often can "read" how you are progressing on your road to recovery.

By helping you with simple tasks, they also assist the hospital staff. Most importantly, caregivers often supply the emotional and physical strength you need but are unable to provide for yourself at this time.

Your caregivers can anticipate your needs and do things to help you feel better. They can read the newspaper to you and talk with you about events that you find interesting. They can locate a program on television or play cards with you. They can surprise you with Popsicles in the afternoon. By keeping you satisfied, occupied and happy, they can help your hospital stay pass more quickly.

Talk about your feelings with your caregivers. Let them help you feel good. Allow them to screen your telephone calls or talk with the medical staff on your behalf. Tell them you appreciate everything they do for you, and don't forget to give your caregivers time to be alone or to go off and do something for themselves. For more on caregivers, see chapter 7.

## Caregivers Need to Take Care of Themselves Too

The biggest mistake caregivers can make is not paying attention to their own needs. Consequently, they may soon discover that their job is an overwhelming and exhausting experience. Because they focus completely on meeting your needs, they may ignore their own well-being — sometimes until it is too late. When this happens, the hospital staff has twice the number of people to worry about — you and your caregiver who is "wiggy" from stress and lack of sleep.

The best way to prevent problems is for caregivers to take time out for themselves every day — even several times a day, if necessary. Caregivers need to be rested, well-fed, alert and feeling good about themselves in order to provide you good care.

Sleeping with a patient in a hospital room sounds nice, but it is not the best idea. Patients are often awake much of the night, and a sleep-deprived caregiver cannot give good care.

Exercise is a good way for caregivers to take a needed break and relieve stress. Walking or jogging around the neighborhood, swimming in a nearby pool and exercising at a local gym are all excellent stress reducers.

## Find Out How to Care for Yourself Before Going Home

Before you are discharged from the hospital, ask to speak with someone on the staff about how best to care for yourself at home. Inquire about the kinds of physical activities you can engage in, what trouble signs to watch for, what professional home-care services may be available to you, and what, if any, dietary guidelines you should follow. In addition, find out who to call if you experience any posthospital problems. Ask to have all this, plus information about any medications you are taking home, put in writing.

Make sure you get a copy of your surgical report (including the anesthesia record) and a list of medications you have been given while in the hospital. Also, ask for copies of your surgical pathology and discharge summary reports.

Take time to fill out any survey forms that come your way. Hospitals can't improve their services unless they get honest feedback from patients like you. Don't be shy about mentioning areas that need improvement — but also sing the praises of those who merit recognition.

Once again, talk with others who have undergone similar procedures about what to expect during your recovery. Just being aware of things you may have to deal with, as well as knowing someone you can talk to, will help allay your concerns as you recover. Here are some other suggestions:

**Expect your recovery not to be as smooth as the medical experts imply.**

If you foresee them, you can navigate rough waters more calmly. Just because yesterday went well, today will not necessarily be smooth sailing. Keep track of your gains each week so you can see your overall improvement.

**Take the pain medication your doctor prescribes for you.**

Don't wait until you are in agony. Anticipate your need for the medication and take it as soon as possible. This will not only allow you to feel much better, but it will enable you to move around and engage in activities beneficial to your healing.

**Don't stay in bed all day.**

Get up and dress each morning — even if just in your sweats. Make yourself a comfortable place to rest during the day in a room other than your bedroom. If this is not possible, then make your bed and lie on top of it with a blanket or coverlet. Try to do a little more for yourself each day. You want to tire yourself enough that you will sleep well through the night. If you must, take short naps during the day, but don't sleep so long that you can't get to sleep at night. Be sure to walk a little every day. Taking your pain medication can really help with this.

## Recognize that medications and your hospital experience can make you depressed.

Don't blame yourself for feeling blue. Acknowledge how you feel and do whatever works to keep your spirits as bright as possible.

## Go slow with eating if you have had any type of abdominal surgery.

Your doctor may tell you that you are free to eat whatever you want. *Do not* take this as encouragement to go all out. Think of your digestive tract as that of a newborn baby and act accordingly. Your digestion will return more to normal, but depending on what was done to you this may take time. Proceed with caution.

## Organize a few friends to assist with your at-home care.

If possible, ask someone to do this for you. If other people are around all day in your household this may not be necessary. However, it is important if you spend more than a few hours alone. You may only need help for a few days, until you regain a greater sense of self-reliance.

In our cases, our husbands were usually at work during the day. We established a system where someone would phone in the morning to assess our needs for the day. Either that same person or someone else would then stop by around midday to visit briefly and deliver groceries or prepared food. Then, in the late afternoon, someone called or stopped by to make sure we were still all right. This routine lasted from three to five days, excluding weekends when family members were around.

## Chapter Thirteen

# How to Stay Sane When Dealing with Insurance Companies

*"In spite of everything that has been reported, the fact is that healthcare today is more comprehensive, accessible and affordable than ever before."*

Stephanie G. Ralphs, President
Comprehensive Medical Connections

We are not experts on all insurance issues. However, we have learned that the more you know about how the system works, and about the specifics of your coverage or any coverage you consider purchasing, the better equipped you will be to deal with whatever situations come your way.

## The Insurance Company Perspective

Make no mistake about it, the number one priority of insurance companies is to make money. This is not to say that insurance carriers are evil or that they don't have your interests in mind. Whether they are set up as for profit or nonprofit corporations, insurance companies must collect enough money to pay claims, support their business activities, and maintain adequate reserves to protect policy holders in the event of insolvency (a requirement mandated by law).

In general, insurance companies get most involved in the most expensive medical decisions. These include hospitalizations, surgeries and lengthy treatment programs. If you belong to an HMO and see your physician for normal outpatient care, your insurance carrier leaves most of the medical decisions up to your doctor and his medical group.

If you belong to a Preferred Provider Organization (PPO) or a traditional healthcare plan, your carrier is sure to be involved in all of your care decisions which are processed as claims. Claims and requests that involve a high dollar amount or which can be considered elective or experimental are certain to be scrutinized closely. This is why documentation of your requests for special treatment is so important.

It is important to realize that insurers are only interested in insuring you to the extent your coverage allows. Make certain that you fully understand the parameters of your policy and, if the policy seems inadequate, augment your coverage while you are still healthy.

Insurance companies are large bureaucracies. Therefore, they have lots of rules and systems and are highly departmentalized. Everything they do is focused on meeting the needs of the majority. This means that they are not set up to respond to a lot of individual exceptions. However, once in a while exceptions do occur. Occasionally, an individual's needs require more or different treatment than is available through standard pathways. Although the climate for dealing with these exceptions within insurance companies is changing, it presently requires extra effort on your part to make beyond-the-norm considerations happen.

Finally, remember that health insurance bureaucracies can appear to move at a snail's pace when responding to issues that are important to you. Sometimes this perception may be real, but in many cases it is merely the anxiety associated with waiting for any kind of insurance company approval, which tends to intensify your feelings of fear and frustration.

# Nine Tips to Help You Navigate the Maze

As hard as we have tried, we still haven't figured out how to wave a magic wand and have all our insurance problems disappear. In the absence of easy solutions, how can you navigate the insurance maze yet retain your sanity? Here are nine tips:

## 1. Secure the very best insurance coverage available while you are still healthy.

Many people make the mistake of not trying to obtain health insurance until after they are diagnosed with an illness. This can be difficult and costly. If you are already ill, this advice comes too late to be of much benefit to you. Even if it is too late for you, give your friends and loved ones a "heads up" message.

Once you have insurance, hang on to it, regardless of your employment or personal situation. Always elect to continue coverage under COBRA or whatever program is available to you.

Consider your lifestyle and long-term plans when choosing an insurance program. Think about what you plan to be doing in the next five to ten years. Do you intend to travel, and therefore need a flexible and large pool of doctors to chose from? If so, perhaps a PPO would be best suited to your needs. Do you intend to remain in your current city, and are you most concerned about the cost of insurance coverage? Then perhaps an HMO is the way to go. In many cases, you will have options. Make the effort to identify the one best suited to you.

## 2. Thoroughly understand your coverage before getting hot under the collar.

Educate yourself before you get sick. Read all the literature provided by the insurance company, your employer, your union, or the other entity that issued your policy. Every customer has the right to ask the carrier for a sample contract. Do so and read it carefully. Then review the lists of doctors and hospitals available to you under the plan. Make certain you are comfortable with your list of available choices.

You cannot expect your insurer to cover you for benefits that aren't in your plan. If your coverage is not comprehensive, explore ways to increase your benefits.

### 3. Understand your carrier's rules and timetable for issuing approvals.

Most carriers have established schedules for processing requests and paperwork. They follow their guidelines, not yours. Find out in advance what these are.

Generally, the more serious the condition, the shorter the time frame for approval; the more elective the procedure, the longer the time frame. Unless it is a life-or-death situation, don't frustrate yourself by trying to schedule a CT scan for the day after tomorrow if your carrier requires four working days for approval. You will end up beating your head against a very thick wall. The same applies if you request approval too early. You might know two months prior to surgery that you are going into the hospital. You might think your insurance carrier would appreciate this information well in advance — wrong! Insurance companies review requests on a set schedule, such as four weeks in advance. If your notification arrives eight weeks before your surgery date, it will sit in their holding file until four weeks out, when their official review process begins. Calling to ascertain your status prior to the initialization of a review will get you absolutely nowhere.

Generally speaking, most contracts state that it is the member's responsibility to obtain proper approvals for procedures. Your physician may offer to take care of this for you. For routine matters, this is probably fine, but for major things it doesn't hurt to call your carrier yourself, just to make sure the proper processes and time frames are being observed.

If you follow all of your carrier's rules and your request is still denied, then by all means appeal the decision. Insurance companies will respond reasonably to such requests. For example, if your primary care physician refers you to a specialist and, before seeing that doctor, you call to confirm that he participates in your insurance plan, your carrier will usually authorize the claim even if it turns out the specialist was not on your list of authorized providers.

### 4. Learn the steps in the approval process.

Find out how the systems for approvals and physician referrals work. Call up the member services department of your insurer and ask the personnel to walk you through your coverage, including how to get authorization for hospitalizations, tests and other procedures. Some companies have this information outlined in written form. If so, ask them to send you a copy and read it cover to cover.

When you call to notify your carrier about an upcoming procedure, ask the representative to tell you everything that will happen in consideration of your request. Does a processor write up the request? Who reviews it? Will a doctor be involved in the evaluation? How many days will it take? At what point are you able to provide more information, if necessary? How will you know whether your request has been approved? Ask all of your questions up front and document in writing everything you are told. Include the name of the person you talked to and the date and time of your call. This information would be critical, should you ever want to appeal a decision.

## 5.  Find out how to get a decision changed.

Ideally, you want to head off any challenges to your request before a denial is issued, but it is a good idea to be prepared in case you need to file an appeal.

Your insurance company generally looks at three criteria when reviewing decisions: whether the procedure is medically necessary, whether your policy covers the procedure, and whether you are eligible to receive the benefit because your premiums are paid up. An insurer is more likely to change a decision if you can demonstrate that what you are asking for is medically necessary. You may be able to accomplish this simply by providing a letter of explanation from your doctor. Also provide your carrier with any published articles and research documentation that back up your request. The more material you have to substantiate your claim, the more likely your carrier is to listen to you. Make sure you ask what your insurer's time frame is for reviewing your appeal, so you know when to call if you have heard nothing.

If you have done all of the above and still feel that your voice is not being heard, consult a good attorney who handles health insurance issues. This is not to say you should use "potential legal action" as leverage to threaten your insurance carrier. Save your big guns for the really big battles.

### 6. Act like a professional.

Dealing with a bureaucracy can be incredibly frustrating. Don't let the process get to you. Ask your questions and conduct yourself in a cordial, businesslike manner. You want your carrier to perceive you as an intelligent, thoughtful, well-intentioned citizen, not a wigged-out, emotional basket case. In the long run, behaving like a professional will get you more positive results.

Prepare for a telephone call to your insurance representative as you would for any important meeting. Organize your thoughts, write down your questions, be very specific with regard to your request. Have all pertinent information at your fingertips — this includes your policy and ID numbers, your doctor's name, the date of the procedure in question and any authorization number assigned to your request.

It is true that the squeaky wheel gets the grease. Don't be shy about repeatedly following up on your request. Be persistent (but professional, of course!) until you get the response you want.

### 7. Find an advocate.

Find someone who will go to bat for you with your insurance company. Your goal is to find a person who can help you move the process along. This can be the insurance broker through whom you obtained your policy, someone at your place of employment or union, or even a person who works for your carrier. Generally, the higher up the chain of command this person is, the better.

### 8. If the stress of handling your insurance matters is too much, assign the duty to someone else.

Sometimes the stress of handling your own insurance matters is too much to endure. Before you get to this point, assign the responsibility to someone else. Find someone who is well organized, pays attention to detail, is able to handle stress, makes a positive impression (at least over the telephone), holds your best interests at heart and is persistent. This can be your spouse, an adult child, a close relative, a trusted advisor or even your insurance broker.

**9.  Obtain copies of what your doctor writes about you and sends to your insurers.**

If you are on any form of disability, insurers from time to time ask doctors to fill out forms to update them on your medical situation. When such a request is issued you should get a copy of the letter, or your carrier may send the forms to you and ask you to forward them to your doctor. Ask your doctor for a copy of her response. These requests are usually fill-in-the-blank forms that do not include your doctor's notes of specific office visits. They are good for you to have on hand for at least two reasons. First, reading them can help you to know if you and your doctor are in agreement regarding your state of health. In addition, your insurer uses these forms to help evaluate your ongoing disability status. The people reading these forms look for descriptive phrases which help them determine things like your ability to resume some form of work. If you disagree with what your doctor has written about your situation or feel that her responses are not descriptive enough, then the sooner you and your doctor address the issue the better.

## Long-Term (Custodial) Care

None of the healthcare plans available today offer long-term custodial care. It must be purchased as a separate policy, which is priced according to your age at the time of purchase. The premiums are fixed for the term of the policy. We strongly recommend that you purchase a long-term plan while in your fifties, because to qualify you must go through an underwriting process and could get turned down if you wait until you are much older or become sick. Waiting too long to take this action could place a devastating financial burden on you and your family.

## Healthcare Reform and What It Means to You

Healthcare reform has been a hot topic for over a decade, and much legislation has been enacted requiring insurance carriers to be more responsive to consumer needs. Three federal laws that provide benefits to healthcare consumers are:

- **COBRA,** the Consolidated Omnibus Reconciliation Act of 1985, allows consumers holding group insurance through their employers to leave their jobs and continue to receive the same health coverage by paying for it themselves. This is advantageous because you do not have to requalify medically for the policy. COBRA allows you a comfortable period of at least eighteen months to decide whether you want to purchase an individual plan through the same carrier or obtain new insurance through a new employer.
- **HIPAA,** the Health Insurance Portability and Accountability Act, or Kennedy-Kassebaum Act. became effective on July 1, 1997. It requires insurance companies who sell small-group and individual plans to offer people "portability" in their health insurance coverage. This means you can now move from one group insurance plan to another within the same company, or from a group to an individual plan, without having to requalify. This is especially important for people with pre-existing conditions.

  As with all federal regulations, there are rules that must be followed to ensure eligibility under these two acts. Some important ones to remember are that if you leave your employer, you must sign up for COBRA at that time; and you must exhaust your COBRA benefits before you can qualify for HIPAA. Understanding and following these rules is critically important to people who might not qualify for coverage under the normal underwriting process, including those who are seriously ill or have pre-existing conditions.
- **Medicare** is available to those sixty-five and over, as well as anyone under that age whom the federal government certifies as being disabled. Its coverage has been expanded in 1998, and those eligible will suddenly find they have many more program options. Participants will be able to choose from traditional indemnity types of plans, HMOs or PPOs. There are benefits to each, and each person must thoroughly examine and understand each plan to determine the best option.

Many senior HMO programs supported by Medicare exist across the nation. These programs often provide a high level of coverage for a zero monthly premium.

Many states are enacting laws to supplement and broaden national healthcare legislation. Be sure to check on consumer-friendly legislation now in effect in your state. Here are two examples of recent California reforms:

- While federal COBRA has been around for almost twenty years, it only protects individuals working at companies with twenty or more employees. The **CAL COBRA** law now extends this protection to those working for companies with two or more employees.

- California's small-group health insurance law, **AB1672**, essentially guarantees coverage to many consumers who were previously unable to obtain health insurance by preventing insurance companies from denying health plans to small businesses due to the health status (serious illnesses or pre-existing medical conditions) of their employees. It also protects these small businesses from high rate increases because of the medical claims of their employees. Cost increases are now capped at ten percent above standard rates for the same coverage.

Healthcare reform has meant good news for consumers, and prospects are excellent for even more far-reaching changes in the future. We encourage you to pay attention to what's happening with regard to healthcare legislation in the news, and to make your opinions heard by voting for legislators who are working toward ways to make the system better for all consumers.

## Insurance Information Resources

More independent resources are becoming available to help you work through your insurance issues. Your first inquiries should be directed to your employer, union, or the organization through which you obtained your policy, but other resources may be available through your local hospital, medical center or social service agency. Many of these now have patient resource centers focused on serving a wide range of patient needs. Two other resources, are **Comprehensive Medical Connections** (800-564-6467), which provides free advice regarding health insurance nationwide; and **HICAP** (415-861-4444), which provides health insurance counseling for individuals in California who are sixty-two years and older or receiving Medicare.

# Chapter Fourteen

# Next Steps

*When I finally finished all of my chemotherapy and radiation for lymphoma, people kept asking me, "Aren't you thrilled to be done?"*

*Of course I was thrilled, but there was something nagging at me — a feeling of uncertainty about the fact that I was no longer actively doing anything to keep the disease away. Also, as hard as it had been, I had gotten used to the treatment routine. I was left with a huge void in my life, as well as a horrible radiation cough that kept me awake at night and left me feeling exhausted during the day.*

*I needed to find a way to make my "life after cancer" meaningful and workable.*

Mac

## Now That Your Treatment Is Over

One of your most surprising and disturbing discoveries may be that you tend to feel worse about your situation after your treatment program is over. The realization that your disease could recur is especially frightening. No longer actively combating it only makes you more anxious. Many feel depressed because their world is once again changing. Severing your link with your doctor, who helped you feel more secure about your situation, may give you the sense of being cast into the water without a life vest.

Even if you hated the routine of doctor visits followed by treatments followed by more doctor visits into which your life had evolved, you feel worse now that no one is actively helping to ensure that your illness doesn't return with a fury. While going through the stages of discovery, diagnosis, and active treatment, life as you had known it was suspended and had been replaced by a new routine of doctor visits, hospitalizations, and often a quieter tempo. In many cases, other people assumed responsibility for the wide range of activities that once were an important part of your life.

Depending on how long your treatments lasted, you may have become very accustomed to your new situation and its pace. In addition, you started to appreciate all of the supportive and now familiar individuals who played such an important role in your getting well. In many ways they became like a second family to you.

It comes as a real shock when many of these same people suddenly disappear. No longer can you look forward to Tuesdays when you paid a regular visit to your doctor's office, or to Fridays at 11:00 A.M. when you had a standing appointment with the lab technician who drew your blood. In addition, visits from friends and personal caregivers slow down or stop altogether now that your crisis is over. For some of us, this new development seems almost worse than the discovery that we were sick.

The many resources that were available to you while you were sick do not carry over into this new, supposedly healthy phase. Emotionally, you are left to go over the falls without even a barrel.

We hope that healthcare professionals will come to recognize the importance of this post-treatment phase in the recovery process and will begin to establish support mechanisms to more easily assist a patient's return to a normal lifestyle. Until these exist, here are some of our own homegrown suggestions:

### Acknowledge how you feel.

Be honest with yourself about how you feel. It is perfectly reasonable for you to be depressed and to sense a huge void in your life at this point. You've been through a heck of a lot, and although you may never have thought you would end up feeling like this, accept that it is okay.

### Seek help.

Find someone with whom you can share your feelings. If you have a spouse, share your thoughts with him or her. You may be surprised to find that they, too, have some of these same feelings. Spouses, because they often walk the same road that you do and feel your pain almost as much as you, can also develop similar feelings of depression and abandonment.

Your friends may no longer know how to help you now that your treatments are over. Be open with them about what you are going through and keep them in your life by enjoying activities together. Let them know that, even though your treatments are over, you are still going through a process of recovery and that you appreciate their patience and support.

Consider joining a support group where the focus is on post-treatment needs and recovery. More and more of these types of groups are being started all over the country. If none of the above suggestions seem to help, seek a professional therapist who can help you sort out and deal with your feelings.

### Develop a new routine.

Just because your daily routine has been forcibly changed doesn't mean you can't develop a new and equally satisfying one. Take pleasure in designing new ways to spend your days. Incorporate the best of your old routines and add new experiences into the equation. Recognize that, even if you could go back to the way things were, they wouldn't be the same because you are no longer the same.

If the end of treatment means that you are able to discontinue the use of certain medical devices, physical therapy aids or things like chemotherapy wigs and hats, have some fun by inviting your close friends over for a party to celebrate. Bury the wigs in a mock ceremony and toast your friends with champagne as a way of saying thank you for their support. Donate your old walkers, canes, or wheel chairs to a community organization or a friend who may now need them. Use what you have learned from your illness experience to fashion an interesting and satisfying new life.

## Use visualization to create a positive mental image.

Employ this technique every day to keep your energies focused on staying happy and feeling well. Combine this practice with a relaxation or deep breathing exercise to maintain your emotional balance.

## Adjust your life.

There may be physical differences between what you used to do and now. Instead of allowing these differences to get you down, find productive ways to adjust your life. For example, if you suffer from heart problems and can no longer race in marathons, find an exercise routine that offers at least some of the benefits of your old one without putting you in physical danger. Don't focus on all of the things that you are no longer able to do. Instead, explore new ways to bring similar satisfaction. If you used to play singles tennis, try doubles. If you must adhere to certain dietary restrictions, take the opportunity to try out new foods and recipes. You may not be able to change the fact that you must now live a more restricted life, but you can choose how you react to it.

*After I was put on three different medications for cardiomyopathy, the congestive heart failure I had been experiencing cleared up. When I asked my doctor about exercise, he recommended that I participate in a cardiac rehabilitation program at my local medical center. This twelve-week program began with full monitoring of my heart during exercise. I learned to recognize when I was putting too much stress on my heart, so I could adjust my level of activity. At first, I depended exclusively on the heart rate monitor that I wore during any vigorous activity. Now, I have more trust in my body and a good sense of what my heart can take. I walk three miles daily, play doubles tennis regularly, have hiked between mountain towns in Italy and even worked to save my vacation house from flooding by bailing water and filling sandbags. No heart expert would have urged me to go out and engage in all of these activities, but with some adjustment, training and experience, I still enjoy an active lifestyle much as I did before.*

Mary

### Give yourself time to adjust.

Aside from your emotions, you may also be experiencing longer-term effects of treatment, such as fatigue, pain, coughing or digestive problems. It will take time and some adjustments to your routine to get you back to feeling well. This is normal. Don't push yourself unreasonably through this process. Keep in mind that "normal" now may be somewhat different than before.

### Reset your priorities.

Now is the time to really think about your priorities. While you were going through your diagnosis and treatment, you may have made some promises to yourself such as, "If I get through this, I promise to quit smoking," or "I pledge to get more exercise." Review these promises and decide whether you intend to fulfill them. Then start making a plan to carry out your commitment.

You also may have made some beneficial changes to your daily routine while you were ill. Perhaps you reduced your level of activity and allowed time for reading, relaxing, listening to music, and really appreciating friends. If any of these changes brought more meaning and satisfaction into your life, continue them now that you are on the road to recovery.

If you were working and took extended time off to concentrate on your treatment, assess whether jumping back into the same environment is best for you. Now is the time to explore other options. Even if you are anxious to pick up where you left off, realize that things will never be completely the same. You have changed as a result of your experience and the people and the environment you once knew may have changed as well. Be open to looking at your old situation with new eyes.

### Set goals and make plans.

The best way to keep healthy and focused on the future is to give yourself things to look forward to. Set new goals and make plans to reach them. Start small and choose goals that have real meaning for you — not just to satisfy others. Maybe you would like to get physically stronger. Start out by walking around the block. If once around is all you can do, be happy, and then write out a plan to gradually increase your level of activity. Don't expect to climb a mountain tomorrow. Don't sign up to run a marathon unless you really want to.

Set your sights on events and goals that you look forward to. Mark them in your calendar and review it weekly. Imagine yourself living those goals. Perhaps you want to visit Europe in the spring or have your grandson visit you over the holidays. Visualize yourself touring Paris or playing catch with your grandson. Keep these images in your mind until you make them a reality.

If you would like to read more about life after treatment, we recommend *Dancing in Limbo: Making Sense of Life After Cancer,* by Glenna Halvorson-Boyd and Lisa K. Hunter.

## Here We Go Again: How to Deal with Recurrences

Wouldn't it be wonderful if you had only one encounter with a serious illness, got cured quickly, and never had to deal with it again? Unfortunately, this is not always the case.

Many of us have to deal with recurrences, new diseases, chronic illnesses and the permanent aftereffects of treatment. When any of these occur, it can seem that not only has your body betrayed you, but so have all the things you employed to get through the earlier crises. The wish to give up is never so acute. If you felt like crawling into a hole and giving up before, these feelings are multiplied the second, third and fourth times around.

Both of us have reached this point several times. It is not a fun place to be, but we are living proof that you can hit the mat more than once and get up swinging. Here are some strategies that have worked for us:

### Don't assume that your time is up.

Just because you have a recurrence or have been diagnosed with a new disease does not mean you are going to die as a result. There is no rule that says we are dealt only two cards in life. Don't give in. Apply the same courage and strength now that you did in your previous situation.

**Remind yourself that a good strategy can work.**

Even though you're back where you started, remember that you have successfully faced these challenges before, and you can do it again. In fact, the next time around might be easier because you are now familiar with a lot of what's involved. Use the knowledge and skills you acquired from your first experience to seek information, talk with your doctors, and build your support team.

**Seek new approaches and treatments that may be available.**

New developments in medicine happen very quickly. Therapies seem to change almost overnight, and new opportunities for controlling your situation may be right around the corner. Investigate any changes that have occurred since your last experience. Look into the possibility of participating in a clinical trial for treatment of your illness. Many studies are specifically targeted to those with recurrences or advanced disease. In addition, if you didn't try complementary or alternative therapies the first time around, you may want to consider them now.

**Rethink some decisions.**

Look at your current situation with an open mind. If you made some choices about treatments and procedures the first time around, you may want to revisit those decisions in light of your recurrence. Facing an illness for the second time often makes us more pragmatic. For example, you may have refused an earlier recommendation to have a permanent colostomy. If this now becomes a key factor in keeping you alive, you might want to change your mind. The same applies to transplants or treatments that will permanently affect your way of life.

**Talk with others who have gone through the same experience.**

You may be surprised at how many others have lived through similar situations. Find out who they are and make a point to talk with them. Ask them how they coped and use any ideas that fit your own situation. Pay attention to non-verbal clues. Do these people seem to have a fighting spirit? Have they found humor to be an effective aid? Connecting with others who share your plight can really help to ease the pain. In addition, their success strategies may be just the antidote that you need to succeed in your current battle.

# Chapter Fifteen

# Facing Death

*Things were not going well for me in 1995. My cancer kept returning, swelling my belly, inhibiting my breathing and making digestion an increasingly difficult experience. I kept visiting doctors in hopes that someone would offer me a miracle.*

*"The good news," they would always say, "is that your cancer is a slow-growing one." What they wouldn't discuss is that fact that it kills just the same.*

*It was a frightening and frustrating few months. Everywhere I went, everything I did was a struggle. Finally I just accepted the fact that I was going to die by the end of the year. With this point of view came the sudden urge to make certain my affairs were in order. This wasn't just a passing notion. I was consumed by it. Not only did I think about it day and night, I talked about it too. My poor husband! I nearly drove him crazy with questions regarding my estate and what he was going to do "after I was gone." I became convinced and excited that my dying would somehow benefit him!*

*I talked about my dying with absolutely everybody — my family, my friends, my oncologist, nurses, casual acquaintances and even perfect strangers. From talking, I moved on to action. I reviewed my will, organized all my files and documented where everything was. I even wrote my obituary, notes to my loved ones and detailed instructions for my memorial service. I felt compelled to "dot every i and cross every t."*

*All this took me several weeks to accomplish. I think I barely slept during that time. My need to get it all done was overwhelming. I almost felt as if I were being driven by some unknown power.*

*The moment I finished, the most unexpected thing happened. An incredible feeling of peace and completion came over me and stayed. Miraculously, my perspective had changed. Although I still believed I was going to die, I no longer viewed it as a frightening outcome.*

*What interested me now was to focus, not on extending my life, but on living it to the fullest. I felt like I had as a kid on summer vacation, but instead of being bored by the prospect of no schedule, I relished the opportunity to sit back and take in the world. For the first time in a long time I really enjoyed getting to know people. Spending time with my family and good friends was pure joy. Taking the time to talk one-on-one with people to whom I previously wouldn't have given the time of day spurred me to open my eyes to new ideas and outlooks. I could now sit in my garden for hours and just marvel at all of the beautiful things I was seeing for the first time. It was clear to me that when I stopped focusing on "doing," I started to understand what it really means to live.*

Alice

## The Time to Put Your Affairs in Order Is Now

There comes a time in each of our lives when it is prudent to put our affairs in order. The time to consider and take care of this is when you are feeling well. If you put off this task until it becomes an absolute necessity, the burden may be overwhelming, and you may lack the clarity of thinking necessary to make important decisions. We hope you have already planted the financial seeds necessary to allow your loved ones to live comfortably in your absence. Now, by making the effort to think about and organize your personal and financial affairs, you will be able to sleep better, knowing you have done everything in your power to look after the interests of those you love.

Putting your affairs in order need not be a morbid or depressing exercise. Far from it. Instead, it can become a stimulating and positive soul-searching experience. Rather than dwelling on your death, focus on the future security and happiness of your family. Clarify what is really important to you and find a way to deal with critical issues. Creating a plan goes a long way toward easing the tensions and frustrations that arise when loved ones don't know what to do following your death. Believe it or not, taking care of all of this when you feel well can actually evoke an incredible feeling of freedom.

Here are some practical tasks you may need to address.

**Make out your will.**

A properly executed will ensures that your wishes will be carried out with a minimum of confusion. Include provisions not only for the major portions of your financial estate, but also for the distribution of personal mementos, instruments, autos, clothing, china, art, jewelry, and even your personal papers. Arguments over these "little things" can really drive a family apart. If you want your trombone to go to your daughter Susan, make sure you clearly state this in your will.

**Seek professional advice.**

Talk with an attorney who specializes in wills and estate planning. Don't try to cut expense corners on this. If cost is of concern, make certain that you prepare in advance for your meeting by completing the steps outlined below. Don't make the mistake of trying to save on the front end by avoiding hiring an expert, and end up causing your family years of tax or other financial problems.

**Locate all of your important documents and make certain they are secure and up-to-date.**

Note the location of each document, and the names and phone numbers of all important contacts. Here is a list of at least some of the items you should keep track of:

1.  *Your will* — Even something in your own handwriting is better than nothing, but a well-drawn will can save your heirs time and thousands of dollars in taxes.

2.  *Medical directives* — These include Durable Powers of Attorney for Healthcare, a Living Will, and any written directions you have for your physician.

3.  *Certificates* — These include your birth certificate and those of your children, adoption certificates, marriage certificates, divorce decrees and your citizenship papers (if applicable), as well as your passport.

4.  *Bank/brokerage/credit account records* — Include all checking, savings, credit, and any other type of account you have with a bank, credit union, savings and loan, or brokerage. Record the passwords and PINs for all accounts and the location of all keys for safe deposit boxes, etc.

5.  *Title records and real property deeds* — These identify you as the owner of any type of valuable property including autos, real estate, recreational vehicles, etc.

6.  *Insurance documents* — Any policies you hold pertaining to health, disability, social security, life, property, auto, homeowners insurance, and any other type of specialized coverage.

7.  *Records of investments and liabilities* — Included with these should be copies of any business and partnership agreements.

8.  *Personal agreements* — These include things like pre-nuptial, guardianship, and trust agreements.

9.  *Retirement, pension and annuity records* — Be sure to note who the beneficiaries are of all these items. If you served in the military, make certain that you retain copies of your service and discharge records.

10. *Income tax returns* — Retain copies of returns for at least seven years.

11. *Names of important contact people* — Include the names, addresses and telephone numbers of your attorney, estate executor, accountant, banker, investment advisor, physicians important to your care, employer pension plan contact, and all other individuals involved in your personal and financial affairs.

Many books have been written to guide you more precisely through this task. Look for them in any bookstore or on the Internet.

Summarize your important information and give copies to your lawyer and a responsible loved one.

Include instructions regarding disposition of your personal writings and papers. If you want them passed on, specify to whom. Give instructions about what to do with your computer files and give any passwords to the person you want to direct this task. Make duplicates of all keys, label them, and keep them in a safe place. Record the codes to any combination locks that secure your personal effects.

## Provide access to ready cash.

If you are the main financial provider for your family, then make sure your loved ones have access to whatever cash they may need between the time that you die and the time your estate is settled.

## Plan your memorial service and write out your wishes.

You don't have to book an appointment with your priest, pastor or rabbi, but you should take the time to commit your wishes to paper. Don't simply mention them casually in passing. Those whom you tell may not take you seriously or remember your requests. In addition, they may have to defend what you told them to other family members, causing needless stress and friction all around.

Do you want a favorite song sung or a special poem read in celebration? Would you like yellow roses or do you prefer white lilies? Do you want to offer a parting message to those who come to your service? Do you even want a service? Don't keep all of this a secret. Those closest to you will feel good knowing that your final tribute will be just as you wished it.

**Write your own obituary.**

Whether or not you expect to have your obituary published, write one anyway. It's not easy to do, but you might get a lot out of it. It may allow you to pat yourself on the back for a life well spent or help you to identify some room for improvement. There's no time like the present to get started doing things that bring real meaning into your life.

**Share your knowledge of family history with younger generations.**

Have someone help you document your family history. Write out a family tree if one doesn't already exist. Tape an oral history of your family, including favorite stories from as far back as you can remember. It doesn't have to be a professionally produced recording. Just talk into the recorder as you remember things. Others can assist you by asking questions about your childhood in order to help jog your memory. This is an especially fun thing to do with the younger members of your family. The point is to not allow yourself to be forgotten, and to leave a legacy that your loved ones can cherish for generations.

*It was not that my affairs were in such bad shape, but once I realized that I had a rare and difficult lung cancer and my time to put things in order might be quite limited, I developed a focused priority that told me to get started now — before my illness or treatment protocol overwhelmed me.*

*For me, the process of getting my affairs in order had four major components. First, I wanted to straighten out my financial affairs, making sure that I was in a good cash position, had brought all documents relative to my beneficiaries up-to-date, and had thought through and prepared both short-term and long-term estate plans.*

*The second item on my list was to resolve my status with my company, with which I had just finished twenty-five good years of creative and fun work. No regrets, but it was definitely time to move on. The complications I had to sort out involved my retirement, which had been planned to take place in only a few months; a post-retirement consulting contract I had already signed; and my complex portfolios of company investments and employee benefits. Resolving these was not an easy task, particularly because the company had changed from the benevolent, founder-run small operation I started with to a large corporation with managers at the top and faceless people below.*

*The third priority was simply to pick up my mess, the piles of papers and boxes of stuff I had been "filing" and saving over years, the many files on work and community projects long past and mostly forgotten. It was good and interesting stuff representing many hours, days, weeks of effort, but all of a sudden it was the past, and I was now dealing only with the present and the immediate future. This was the easiest job — out most of it went!*

*My last, but by no means least priority was to start working again on some things I'd been wanting to complete for several years: my memoirs, family history and travel writings. I wasn't aiming for the great American novel, but I had this feeling that by contemplating and collecting my thoughts and remembrances about my past, and then trying to articulate these thoughts, I could somehow tie my life together at this end. These books might be read and even enjoyed by family and close friends who shared the moments with me, but my main motivation for doing this was me. I wanted to gather the odds and ends of an interesting and exciting life and put them in some kind of order. I decided it would make me feel better and help me focus on the future.*

Wells

## When You Know You Are Dying

At some point in your illness you may come to the realization that a cure is not possible and that you are going to die. This can be a frightening experience for some, while for others it evokes a very freeing emotion. Most of us never really prepare to die; therefore we can find ourselves unprepared to deal with the fear, joy and other ranges of emotions that envelop us and those around us. There is no right or wrong way to approach dying. The important thing is to go through it in the way that has the most meaning for you and your loved ones. Here are some suggestions to ease the burdens associated with dying:

### Acknowledge that you are dying.

Get the subject out in the open. Talk about it with others. Don't make yourself and everyone else go through the experience alone. Lift the cloud of unexpressed emotions that hangs over you and your situation.

### Realize that death experiences are cumulative.

Each death brings back memories of all of the others in our experience. If someone in your circle seems to react to your situation with more difficulty than you think he should, recognize that he may be dealing not only with how he feels about you, but also with unexpressed emotions he has about the loss of other loved ones.

### Validate the emotions of those around you who aren't dying.

You may be the one who is dying, but this is not just your ordeal. Everyone who shares time with you is going through their own emotional experience. Acknowledge their feelings.

### Savor the moments.

Make every moment you have left a precious one. Don't take the same old things for granted. If you see the sun shining, bask in its glow. If the visit of a special friend means a lot to you, share your joy by saying so. You have nothing to lose and everything to gain by sharing your happiness.

### Involve everyone who wants to be involved.

Don't shut people out. Encourage loved ones to participate with you in the time that you have left — especially the children.

### Decide how you want to be cared for and share this information with your doctor and your family.

Don't put loved ones in the position of having to choose how you should die. Talk with your doctor about how you want to be treated and clearly communicate your wishes to those close to you. This will relieve a lot of stress on family members.

**Seek professional help to express all of the emotions you are feeling.**
Let a professional help you frame how and what you want to say to those you dearly love.

## Hospice — For Those Who Want the Comfort of Home and a Safe, Supportive Environment

*"You matter to the last moment of your life, and we will do all we can, not only to help you die peacefully, but also to live until you die."*
Hospice founder, Dame Cicely Saunders

Hospice is a special kind of care designed to provide comfort and the highest quality of life for people in the final phases of a terminal illness. Hospice concentrates on controlling pain and symptoms and teaches family members how to care for the patient as well as how to cope with the emotional, practical, and spiritual concerns related to a loved one's illness.

Hospice services are available to persons who can no longer benefit from curative treatment. The typical hospice patient has a life expectancy of six months or less. Most receive care at home, although hospice services are also available to those who choose to stay in a treatment facility. Services are provided by a team of trained professionals and include palliative care for the patient, counseling to help everyone understand the issues involved in dying and loss, assistance with the completion of family business matters, and funeral plans. Although hospice referrals are usually made by the patient's primary physician, they can come from many sources, such as family members, friends, clergy and other healthcare professionals.

Some hospices also offer a Focused Care Program, which provides both physical and emotional support for families and patients with prognoses longer than six months, as well as for those who want help when facing decisions about treatment choices and medical care.

# Chapter Sixteen

# Are You Taking Charge?

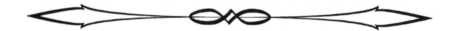

You've made it this far reading this book — congratulations! — but don't stop here. With all you have learned, just think what you are capable of in the management of your illness. Do not feel that you have to incorporate everything we have outlined. Using even a few techniques we discussed will help you better direct your own medical care. Use what works and go from there.

Whether you need to search for information, improve your communications, get organized in general or deal with the emotional ups and downs that come from having a life-threatening disease, this book can help provide you with the knowledge and skills you need.

To decide specifically how you are going to apply what you learned in this book, ask yourself the following questions:

- Am I communicating well with those involved in my healthcare? Have I asked enough questions and gotten the answers? Have I communicated enough about myself and my needs?
- Do I fully understand everything I want to know about my medical condition?

- Am I organized? Do I prepare for doctor visits? Do I have a medical resume and use it? Do I know where my medical records are and how to get them?
- Do I have enough useful information about my situation, and do I know how to find more?
- Are my relationships with my doctors satisfactory?
- Do I have a wellness team that works for me?
- Do I know enough about treatment options that are available to me?
- Do I know why I am taking all my medications, and all the positive and negative effects they could have?
- When I undergo a test or procedure, am I fully aware of what is happening and what the consequences are, both good and bad?
- Will I be prepared for my next hospital stay?
- Am I taking full advantage of the insurance options available to me?
- Are my affairs, personal and financial, in order?
- Am I taking charge?

Consider today a new beginning — one in which you take the best from what life has to offer. Open your mind and heart to new ideas and influences and the support of others. Life is too short to waste time on negative thoughts and actions. Work to effect positive changes in your situation by taking charge of your health and well-being. Best wishes!

# Suggested Reading

Berkow, Robert, M.D., Editor-in-chief. *The Merck Manual of Medical Information—Home Edition*. Whitehouse Station, New Jersey: Merck Research Laboratories, 1997. The world's most widely used medical reference—now in everyday language.

Blau, Sheldon P., M.D., and Elaine Fantle Shimberg. *How to Get Out of the Hospital Alive*. New York: Macmillan, 1997. A guide to patient power.

Capossela, Cappy, and Sheila Warnock. *Share the Care*. New York: Fireside, 1995. How to organize a group to care for someone who is seriously ill.

Cooke, Margaret, and Elizabeth Putnam. *Ways You Can Help*. New York: Warner Books, 1996. Creative, practical suggestions for family and friends of patients and caregivers.

Dollinger, Malin, M.D., Ernest H. Rosenbaum, M.D., and Greg Cable. *Everyone's Guide to Cancer Therapy*. Kansas City: Andrews McMeel Publishing, 1997. How cancer is diagnosed, treated, and managed day to day.

Ferguson, Tom, M.D. *Health Online*. Reading, Massachusetts: Addison-Wesley, 1996. How to find health information, support groups, and self-help communities in cyberspace.

Graedon, Joe, and Teresa Graedon, Ph.D. *The People's Pharmacy*. New York: St. Martin's Griffin, 1996. Your consumer's guide to prescription drugs, over-the-counter drugs, side effects and dangerous drug interactions, home remedies, health and beauty products, and new ways to protect your health at the doctor's office and in the drugstore.

Graedon, Joe, and Teresa Graedon, Ph.D. *Deadly Drug Interactions*. New York: St. Martin's Griffin, 1997. How to protect yourself from harmful drug-drug, drug-food, and drug-vitamin combinations.

Halvorson-Boyd, Glenna, and Lisa K.Hunter. *Dancing in Limbo*. San Francisco: Jossey-Bass, 1995. Making sense of life after cancer.

Landis, Dylan. *Your Health and Medical Workbook*. New York: Berkeley, 1995. The essential health-care organizer for you and your family.

Lerner, Michael A. *Choices in Healing*. Cambridge, Massachusetts: MIT Press, 1994. Integrating the best of conventional and complementary approaches to cancer.

Morra, Marion, and Eve Potts. *Choices*. New York: Avon Books, 1994. A sourcebook for cancer information, from medications and modern therapies to the latest research procedures and diagnostic technologies.

Moyers, Bill. *Healing and the Mind*. New York: Doubleday, 1993.

Murphy, Gerald P., M.D., Lois B. Morris, and Dianne Lange. *Informed Decisions*. New York: Viking Books, 1997. The complete book of cancer diagnosis, treatment, and recovery.

People's Medical Society. *Dial 800 for Health*. Allentown, Pennsylvania: People's Medical Society, 1997. A comprehensive listing of medical, nutritional and general health-related hotlines, services and advice.

Remen, Rachel Naomi, M.D. *Kitchen Table Wisdom*. Riverhead Books, 1996. Stories that heal.

Tyberg, Theodore, M.D., and Kenneth Rothaus, M.D. *Hospital Smarts*. New York: Hearst Books, 1995. The insider's survival guide to your hospital, your doctor, the nursing staff — and your bill.

Weiss, Marisa C., M.D., and Ellen Weiss. *Living Beyond Breast Cancer*. New York: Random House, 1997. A survivor's guide for when treatment ends and the rest of your life begins.

Wolff, Michael. *Your Personal Net Doctor*. New York: Wolff New Media, 1996. Your guide to health and medical advice on the Internet and online services.

# Index

# About the Authors

***Alice MacNaughton Hodge*** was born and raised in the Hawaiian Islands. As the seventh child (and a twin) in a family of eight, Alice learned early on how to face life's challenges with grit, determination and a sense of humor. Both her mother and her maternal grandmother died of cancer at the age of forty-two. Alice is a graduate of Stanford University. She is the former senior vice president, sales promotion, for Emporium Department Stores, and former vice president, marketing, for the San Francisco Newspaper Agency. She retired in 1994 to fight her recurring disease and help others in similar situations. Alice lives in Marin County, California with her husband, Jim, two cats and a golden retriever.

***Mary Halsted Lonergan*** was born in West Virginia, grew up in the Midwest and settled in San Francisco after receiving degrees from Mills College and Stanford University. She has devoted her time to raising two children, running a catering business, actively supporting her community as a volunteer and traveling with her husband, Richard. A survivor of three life-threatening illnesses, Mary understands the importance of taking responsibility for one's health and maintaining a balance in life.

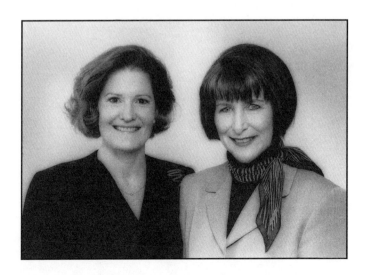

# We want to hear from you!

We welcome your feedback. Tell us what you think about Taking Charge of Your Health. In addition, please include any anecdotes, ideas or suggestions that you may want us to include in our next edition.


Send all feedback to:
Alice Hodge and Mary Lonergan
399 Crown Road
Kentfield, California 94904

or e-mail it to us at:
<Yougetwell@aol.com>

To order additional copies of

# Taking Charge of Your Health

Book: $14.95    Shipping/Handling: $3.50

Contact: ***BookPartners, Inc.***
P.O. Box 922, Wilsonville, OR 97070
Fax: 503-682-8684
Phone: 503-682-9821
Phone: 1-800-895-7323